Fabulous TEEN HAIRSTYLES

A STEP-BY-STEP GUIDE TO 34 BEAUTIFUL STYLES

ERIC MAYOST

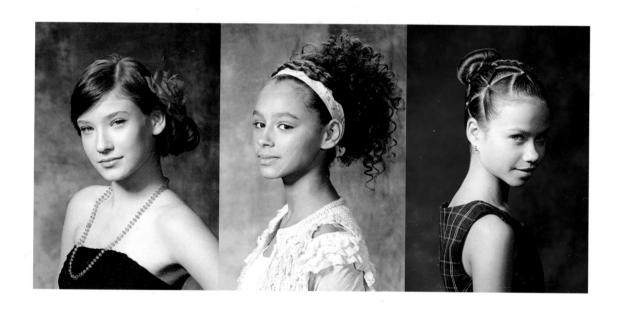

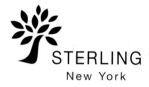

STERLING

New York

STERLING
New York

An Imprint of Sterling Publishing
387 Park Avenue South
New York, NY 10016

Created by Penn Publishing Ltd.
www.penn.co.il

Design and layout by Ariane Rybski
Photography by Roee Fainburg
Edited by Shoshana Brickman
Styling by Louise Bracha
Makeup by Sigal Asraf

ISBN 978-1-4027-8612-9

Library of Congress Cataloging-in-Publication Data

Mayost, Eric.
  Fabulous teen hairstyles / by Eric Mayost.
    p. cm.
  ISBN 9789-8612-4027-1-
  1. Hairstyles. 2. Teenage girls--Health and Hygiene. I. Title.
  TT972.M387 2012
  646.7›240835--dc23

                                    2012018793

Distributed in Canada by Sterling Publishing
c/o Canadian Manda Group, 165 Dufferin Street
Toronto, Ontario, Canada M6K 3H6
Distributed in the United Kingdom by GMC Distribution Services
Castle Place, 166 High Street, Lewes, East Sussex, England BN7 1XU
Distributed in Australia by Capricorn Link (Australia) Pty. Ltd.
P.O. Box 704, Windsor, NSW 2756, Australia

For information about custom editions, special sales, and premium and corporate purchases,
please contact Sterling Special Sales at 800-805-5489 or specialsales@sterlingpublishing.com.

Manufactured in China

2 4 6 8 10 9 7 5 3 1

Contents

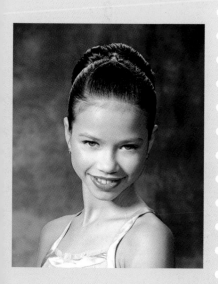

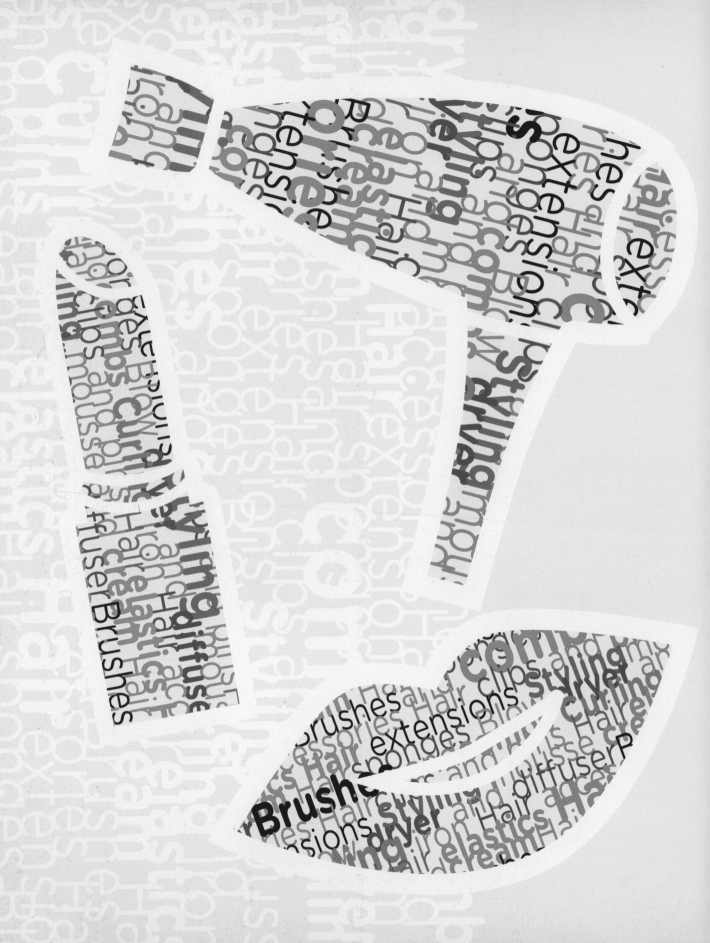

Introduction

Do you love fun hairstyles? Are you getting ready for prom and excited about creating your very own hairstyle and maybe even those of your friends? Want something fancier than a ponytail or braid? Or maybe you know a little girl or tween who loves dressing up or has a fancy occasion on the horizon.

If any of these descriptions sound familiar, then **Fabulous Teen Hairstyles** is just right for you. It's a creative collection of 34 hairstyles designed for today's trendiest girls. All the styles are easy to make in your own home—no specialized training or equipment required. Every hairstyle is accompanied by easy-to-follow instructions, step-by-step pictures, and beautiful photos of the finished hairstyle. You'll find styles for every look and occasion. Glamorously sleek, fabulously fun, charmingly sweet—there's a little bit of everything! Of course, all the styles can be dressed up with coordinating accessories if you like.

With **Fabulous Teen Hairstyles**, you can create a dreamy hairstyle for any special event. Practice a bit first so that when the special occasion arrives, you'll be ready to handle the hairstyle with ease. Save yourself the hassle and cost of rushing out to a fancy hair salon and enjoy the convenience of making the hairstyle that you want, exactly when you want. Of course, it's also terrific hearing compliments about a hairstyle you've styled with your own two hands!

Fabulous Teen Hairstyles is great for teenagers who want to have fun and try their hands at hairstyling. It's also perfect for anyone who wants to style hair for the little girls they love for special parties or events.

About the Author

Eric Mayost has been styling hair since he was nineteen years old. In addition to hairstyling, he has studied art and graphic design. Eric has worked with some of the world's leading hairstylists and has participated in cover shoots for some of the world's leading fashion magazines.

Eric has managed his own hair salon for over a decade and is the author of **Spectacular Hair** (Sterling Publishing, 2010) and **Gorgeous Wedding Hairstyles** (Sterling Publishing, 2012). He has carved a career for himself by creating glamorous hairstyles that stars love, and he enjoys staying at the forefront of hairstyling fashion.

Tools & Accessories

You don't need many tools to create a mini hair salon in your home. I recommend checking to make sure you have everything you need before you start styling. The last thing you want to do is run out of bobby pins just as you are finishing your masterpiece hairstyle!

Blow dryer
Use this to dry freshly washed hair before styling it. In some cases, you'll also need a blow dryer for styling.

Bobby pins and hair pins
These pins are used to secure styled hair in place. In most cases, you'll want the pins to be invisible, so choose ones that match the color of the hair you're styling.

Brushes and combs
You'll need the hair to be tangle-free before you start any hairstyle, so make sure you comb out all the knots first. When you're styling, a round brush is great for creating gentle curls and a paddle brush is just right for increasing volume. You'll also need a tail comb (a.k.a. rattail or fine-tooth comb) to make straight parts and backcomb hair.

Curling iron
Use this to curl the hair. Practice makes perfect when it comes to hair curling, since you want to hold the iron long enough to curl the hair, but not so long that it burns it.

Diffuser
Use this to add volume and accentuate hair that has been curled.

Elastic hair band
This is used to hold hair away from the face.

Hair accessories
Love hair accessories? Who doesn't! You'll find suggestions for hair accessories at the end of many hairstyles, but these are just ideas. Use what you love!

Hair clips

These come in all different sizes and are important to have on hand for holding hair back while you're styling.

Hair elastics

Use these to secure ponytails and braids. Choose ones that are gentle on the hair and don't rip it. In some hairstyles, you'll need really small hair elastics that are visible in the final style. In this case, make sure you choose colors that you like.

Hair extensions

Natural or synthetic hair additions are integrated into hairstyles to add volume and length. Hair extensions may be long or short, round, donut-shaped, straight, or curly. Good quality hair extensions can be reused.

Holding spray

Spray this onto your hairstyle when it's finished to help it last as long as possible. In some cases, you'll want to spray the hairstyle with holding spray during the styling process in order to hold a particular shape. I recommend spraying from a distance of about 8 inches so that the spray is evenly dispersed on the surface of the hair.

Styling mousse

Rub this into wet hair when you need a bit of extra body. It's particularly important when you want to add body and curl to hair that is otherwise straight.

Styling creams

Rub moisturizing cream into dry hair to create a smooth look. Use styling cream for curls when styling curly hair.

Hair sponges

These come in all different shapes and sizes, and are integrated into fancy hairstyles to add body and volume.

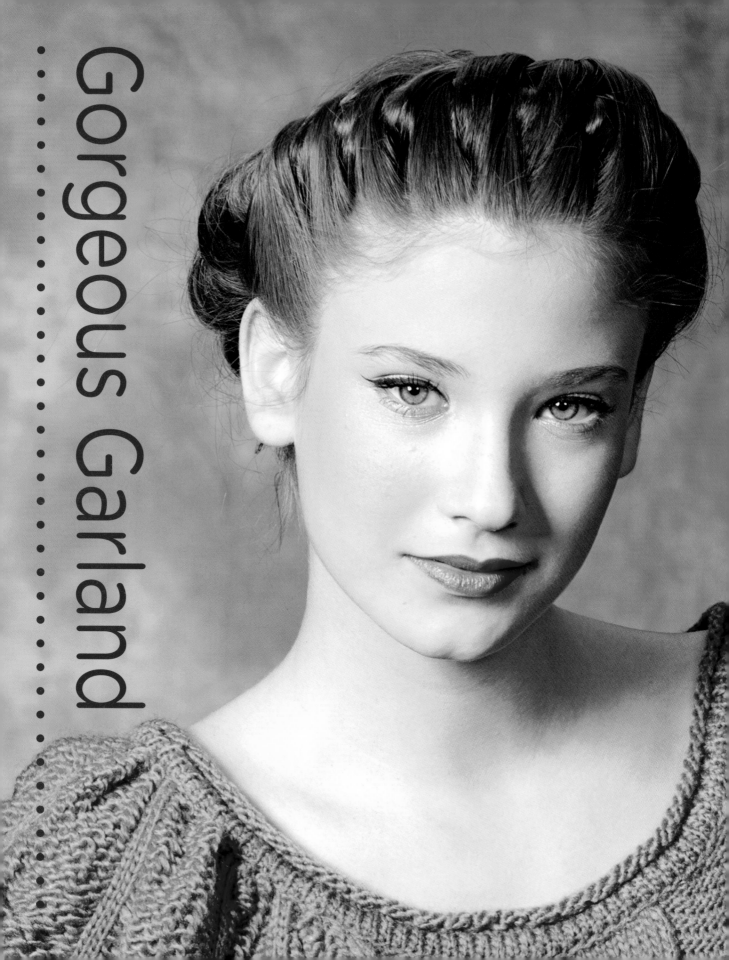

Gorgeous Garland

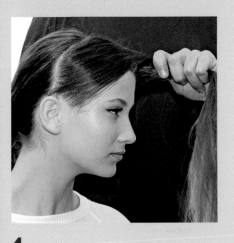

1

1. Wash and blow dry the hair. Make a part that extends from ear to ear over the crown of the head.

2. Grasp a 1-inch section of hair above the right ear.

3. Split the section into two sections and number the sections 1 (closest to the ear) and 2.

4. Bring section 1 over section 2 to make an X and then add a small section of hair from the hairline to section 2.

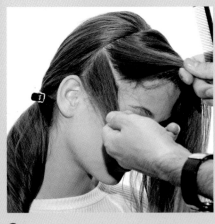

2

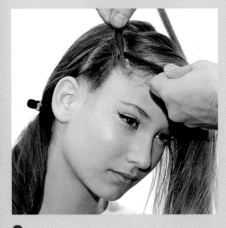

3

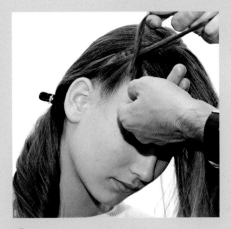

4

Create a natural garland by weaving hair all around the head. Dress up the garland with hair accessories if you like, or leave it stunningly simple.

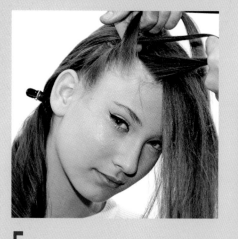

5

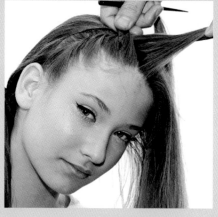

6

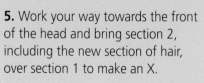

5. Work your way towards the front of the head and bring section 2, including the new section of hair, over section 1 to make an X.

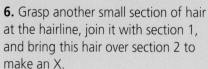

6. Grasp another small section of hair at the hairline, join it with section 1, and bring this hair over section 2 to make an X.

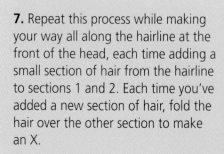

7. Repeat this process while making your way all along the hairline at the front of the head, each time adding a small section of hair from the hairline to sections 1 and 2. Each time you've added a new section of hair, fold the hair over the other section to make an X.

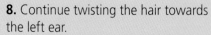

8. Continue twisting the hair towards the left ear.

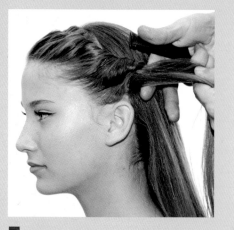

7

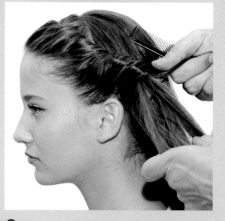

8

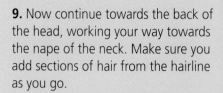

9. Now continue towards the back of the head, working your way towards the nape of the neck. Make sure you add sections of hair from the hairline as you go.

10. Repeat this process around the back of the head. Make sure the garland you are weaving sits a bit higher along the back of the head.

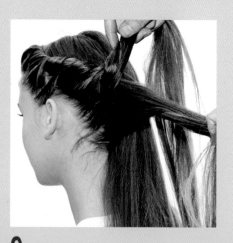

9

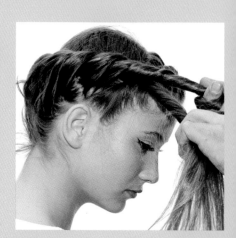

10

11

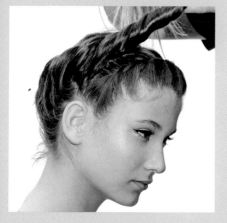

12

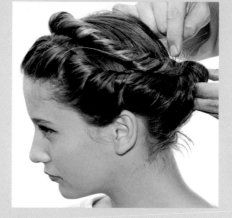

13

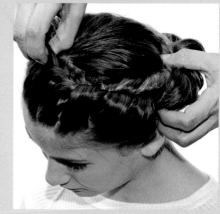

14

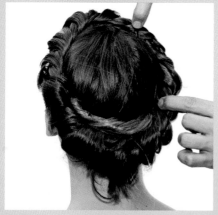

15

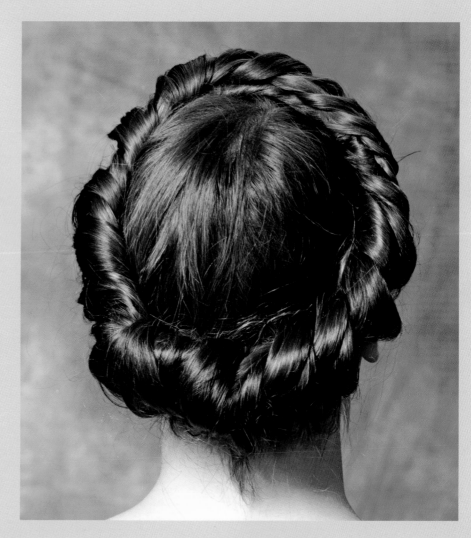

11. When you reach the beginning of the garland and there is no more hair to add from the hairline, twist sections 1 and 2 together.

12. Draw the twisted hair upwards.

13. Wrap the hair around the inner edge of the garland you've just made, tucking it under the garland.

14. Repeat this process until all the hair has been tucked in place.

15. Secure the hair with bobby pins and mist with holding spray.

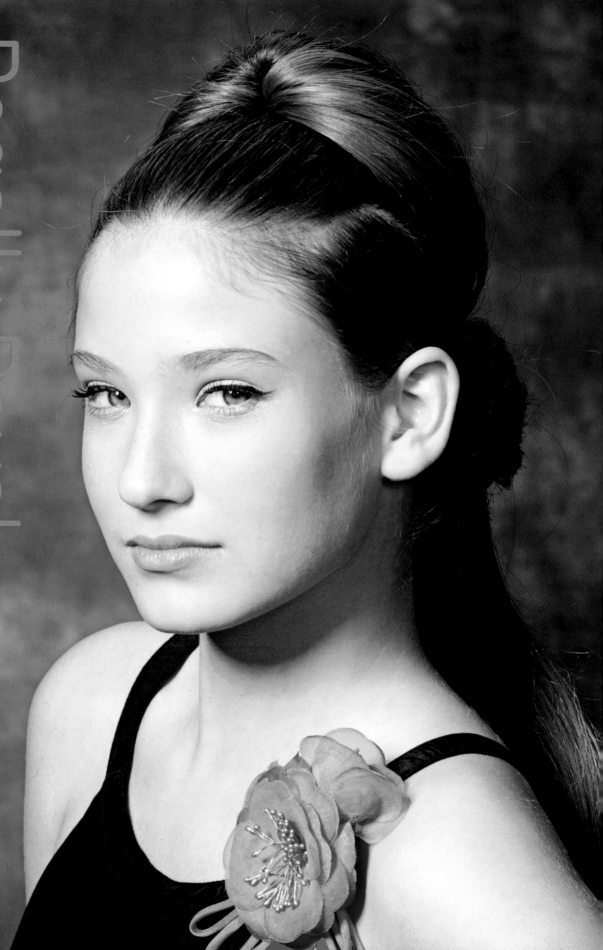

Regally Royal

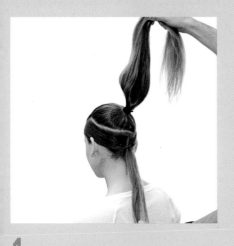

1

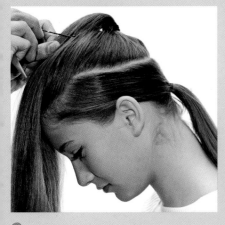

2

1. Wash and blow dry the hair. Separate the hair into top and bottom sections with a round part that runs from above the left eyebrow, around the back of the head, and to the right eyebrow. Secure each section with a hair elastic.

2. Brush the top section of hair forward.

3. Secure this section of hair with bobby pins about 1 inch in front of the hair elastic to create a small bump at the crown of the head.

4. Gently brush the hair in this section backwards and then wrap a hair elastic around the middle of it.

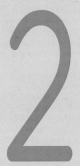

Feeling bold and beautiful? This style is the way to show it! All the hair is drawn backwards, leaving a clean front and dramatic back.

3

4

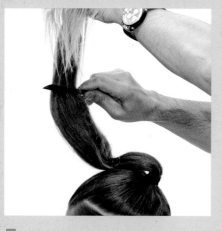

5. Gently backcomb the hair between the hair elastic and the bobby pins you inserted in Step 3 to increase volume.

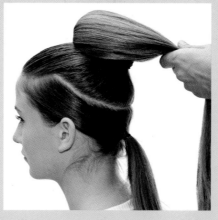

6. Draw this section of hair towards the back of the head, fold it over the bump you created at the top, and bring it over the hair elastic.

7. Brush the top of the hair so that it is smooth and wrap a hair elastic around it, leaving the long ends loose.

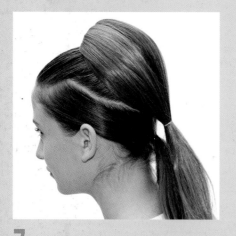

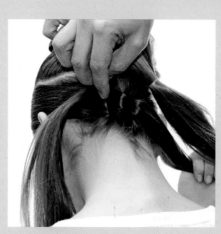

8. Divide the hair in the bottom section into two even sections.

9. Secure these sections on either side of the head with bobby pins.

10. Place the top section of hair between the divided bottom sections and secure it with bobby pins.

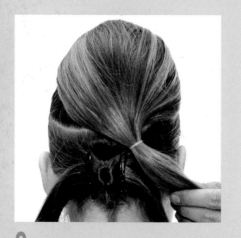

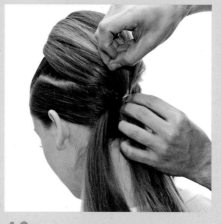

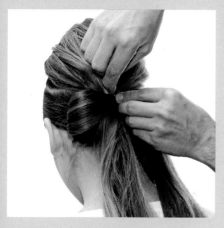

11

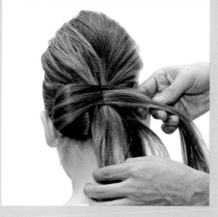

12

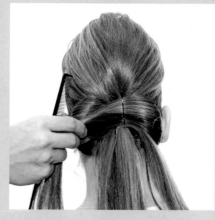

13

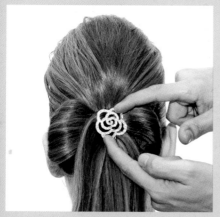

14

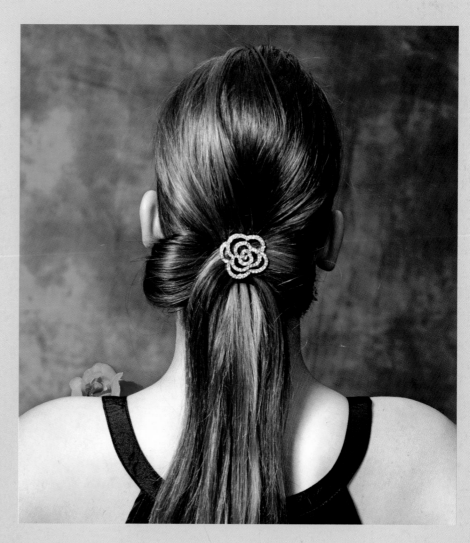

11. Grasp the bottom left section of hair and fold it towards the center.

12. Secure it at the back of the head with bobby pins.

13. Repeat this process with the hair in the bottom right section and secure it with bobby pins.

14. Pin a decorative hair clip at the back of the head to hide the bobby pins and complete the look. Mist with holding spray.

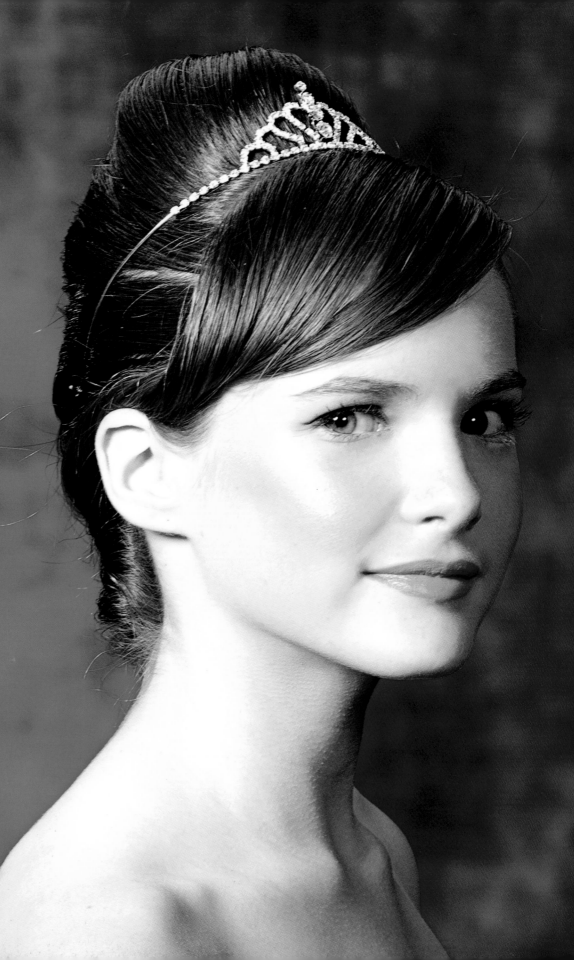

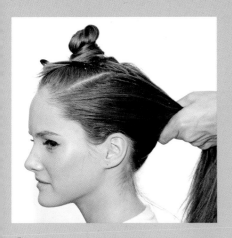

1. Wash and blow dry the hair. Divide the hair into two sections with a part that extends from above the left eyebrow, around the crown of the head and to the right eyebrow. Gather the hair at the crown in a ponytail.

2. Brush the hair below the part to one side and mist with holding spray.

3. Hold the hair at one side of the head, place a brush handle diagonally on the hair, and then wrap the hair over the brush handle and back towards the middle of the head.

4. Roll the hair around the handle to form a twist and secure the rolled hair with bobby pins close to the scalp.

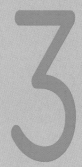

1

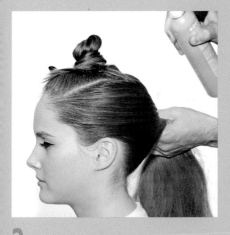

2

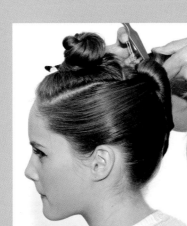

3

4

Create a cornucopia of waves and curls with this design. It looks lovely with a sparkly hair band or tiara, but can definitely be worn unadorned as well.

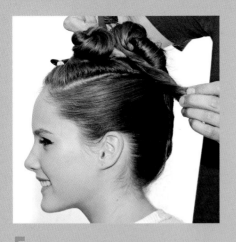

5

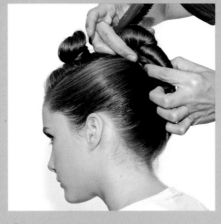

6

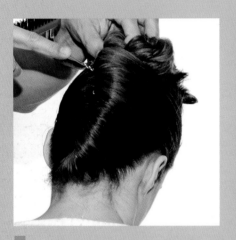

7

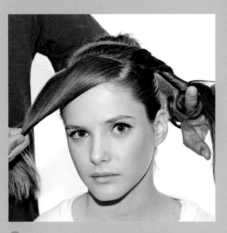

8

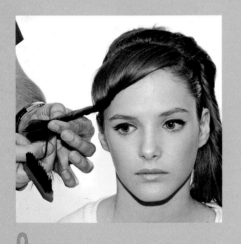

9

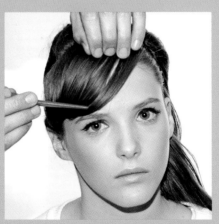

10

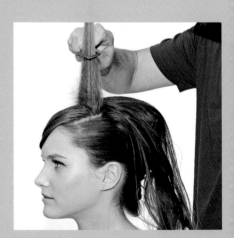

11

5. Carefully draw the brush out of the rolled hair. Make sure you don't ruin the shape of the roll as you do this.

6. Carefully tuck the ends of the hair under the twist again, making sure you don't damage the shape of the twist as you do this.

7. Gently brush the hair so that it is smooth. Insert hair pins along the entire length of the twist to secure it in place.

8. Move to the front of the head and divide the hair into a front and back section.

9. Brush out the front section, hold it at the ends, and twist it towards the forehead. Continue the twist all the way to the ends of the hair.

10. Draw the ends behind the ear and secure them at the base of the larger twist with bobby pins. Adjust the front of the hair so that it looks like there are smooth bangs.

11. Brush out the other section of hair at the front of the head and backcomb the hair at the roots to increase volume.

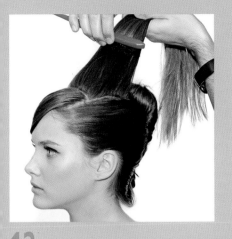

12

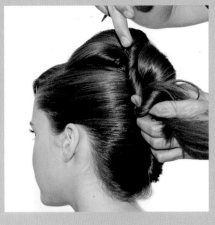

13

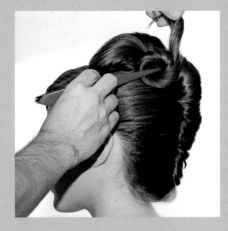

14

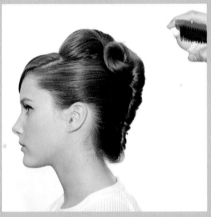

15

12. Gently brush the top of this section as you draw it backwards. You want to brush the hair smooth without reducing the volume.

13. Twist this section of hair, tuck it into the larger twist at the back of the head, and secure with hair pins.

14. Use the end of a tail comb to twist the ends of the loose hair into a loop, and secure the loop with bobby pins.

15. Mist with holding spray.

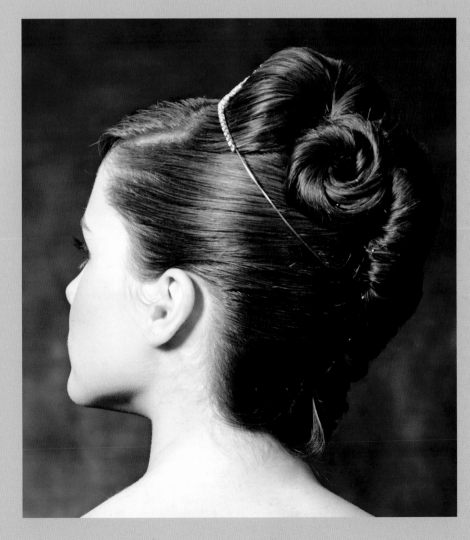

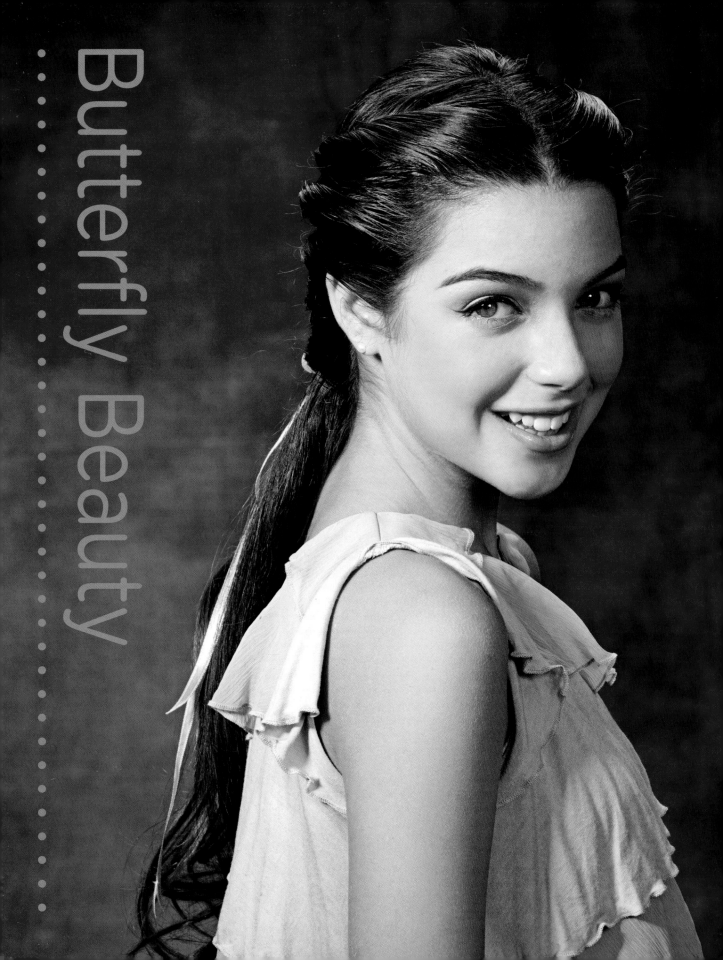

Butterfly Beauty

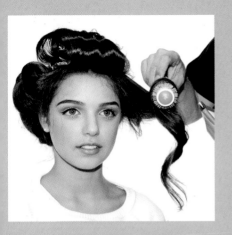

1

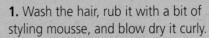

1. Wash the hair, rub it with a bit of styling mousse, and blow dry it curly.

2. Roll every curled section of hair, using a large round brush, and secure the rolls with a clip. If the hair you're styling is quite straight, you may need to make the curls using rollers. Mist with hair spray and wait for about 15 minutes.

3. Gently release the rolls of hair. Grasp a section of hair at the front of the head, to the immediate right of the middle. Twist it inwards and mist with holding spray.

4. Draw the twisted hair to the back of the head with one hand and grasp a small section of hair at the back of the head with the other hand.

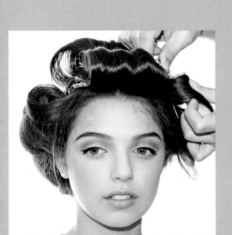

2

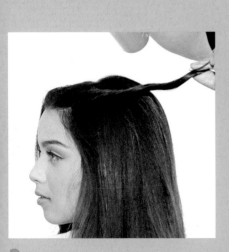

3

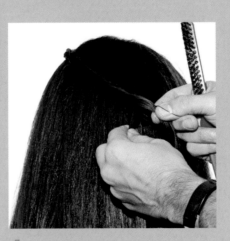

4

This style is just perfect for a beautiful brides-maid of any age. It features a pretty pattern of twisted hair that creates the illusion of butterfly wings.

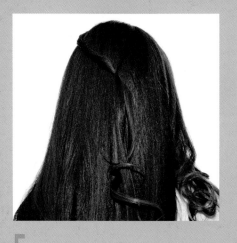

5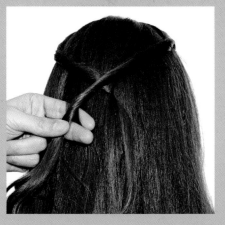

6

5. Connect the two sections of hair with a small hair elastic to secure the twisted section of hair in place.

6. Grasp another section of hair from the front of the head, this time from the immediate left of the middle. Twist it inwards and bring it to the back of the head. Create an X with the first twisted section, drawing it over the hair elastic holding that section of hair to conceal it.

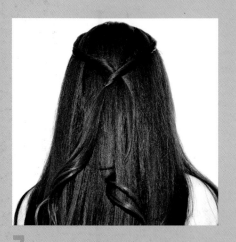

7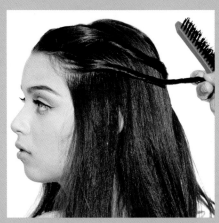

8

7. Grasp a small section of hair from the back of the head and join it with the twisted section of hair you've just drawn backwards. Secure the two sections with a hair elastic.

8. Grasp another section of hair from the front of the head, adjacent to the section you twisted backwards in Step 4, and twist it.

9. Draw the hair to the back of the head and over the second twisted section of hair to form a second X. Secure this section of hair at the back of the head with a hair elastic.

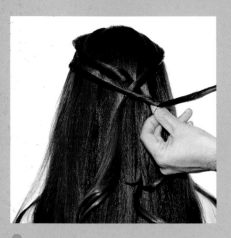

9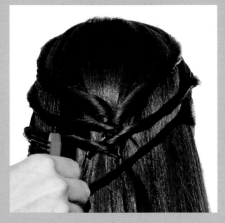

10

10. Continue twisting sections of hair as you draw them backwards, securing them at the back of the head so that they overlap with previous sections of hair.

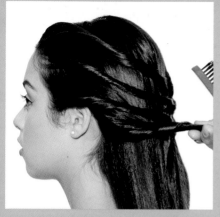

11

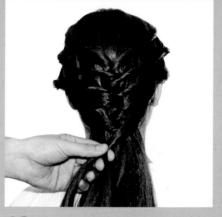

12

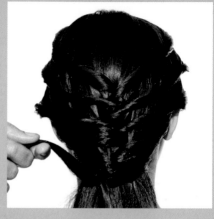

13

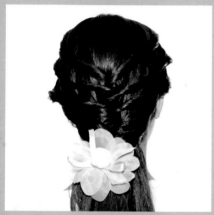

14

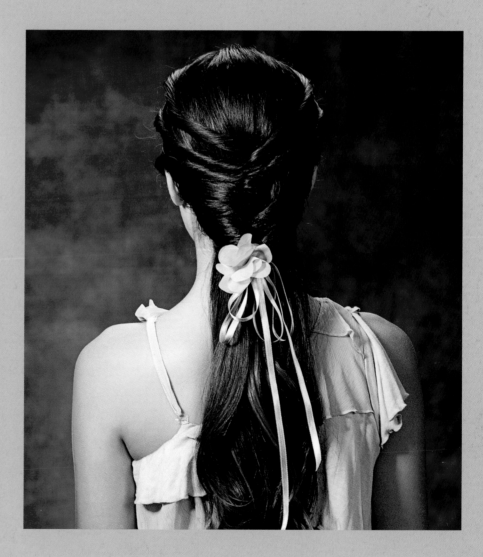

11. Mist each section of hair with holding spray after you form the X-shapes to hold the twists in place and create a clean look.

12. Continue drawing sections of hair backwards like this until you reach the hairline at the back of the head.

13. When you reach the last section of hair, draw it over the last hair elastic to conceal it. Hold this section of hair in place with a hair pin.

14. Mist with strong holding spray Add a pretty floral accessory if you like.

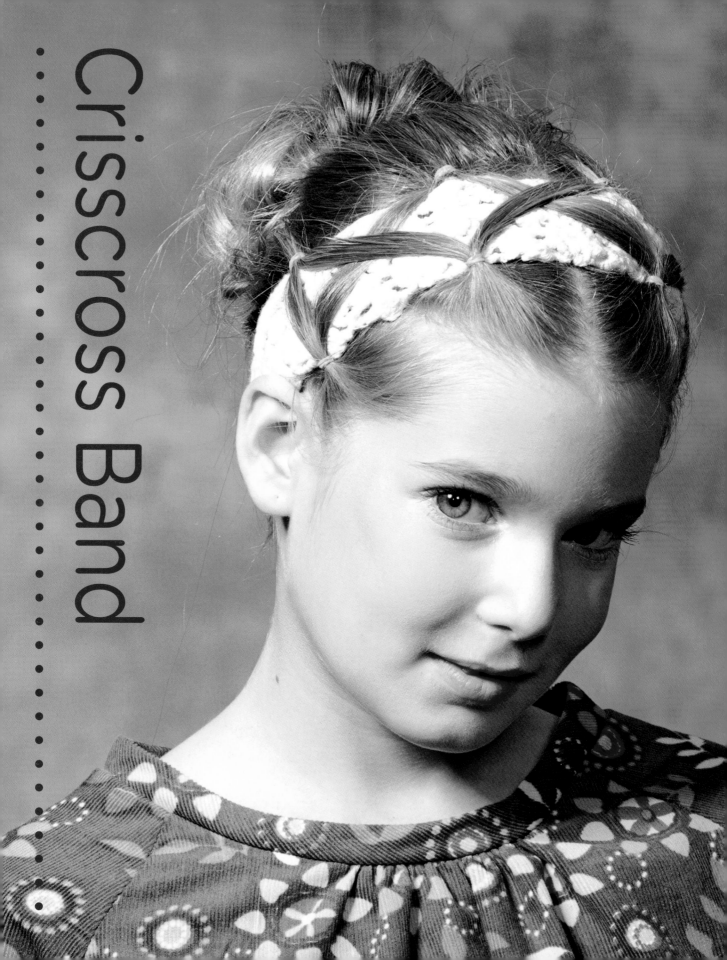

Crisscross Band

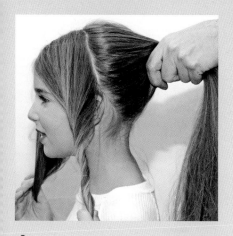

1. Wash and blow dry the hair. Divide the hair into two sections with a part that extends from one ear to the other over the crown of the head.

2. Grasp a small section of hair to the left of the middle of the brow.

3. Secure the hair in a ponytail with a brightly colored hair elastic.

4. Repeat this process to make three more little ponytails, all similar in size, along the hairline.

1

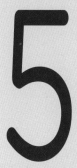

5

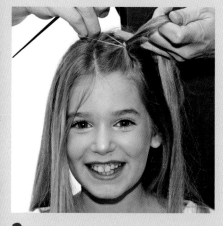

2

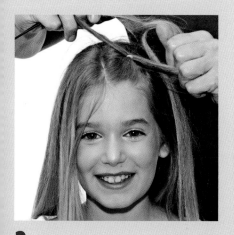

3

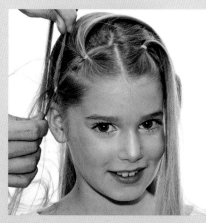

4

Here's a fun design that features an ordinary hair band upgraded with real hair. Make sure you like the hair elastics you choose, since they are visible in the final hairstyle.

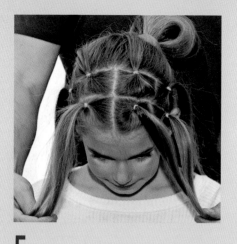

5

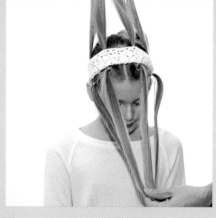

6

5. Make another four ponytails immediately behind the first four so that you have two rows of small ponytails along the top of the head. When securing the second row of ponytails, make sure there is enough room between the two rows of ponytails to place the hair band.

6. Place the headband on the top of the head so that it sits between the two rows of ponytails.

7. Number the ponytails in the first row from 1 to 4. Split ponytail 2 into two even sections.

8. Split ponytail 4 into two even sections. Number the ponytails in the second row from 5 to 8. Draw one section of hair from ponytail 2 and one section of hair from ponytail 4 over the hair band and join them with ponytail 7.

9. Secure these three sections of hair with a hair elastic.

10. Now split ponytail 3 into two even sections. Join one of these sections with the loose section of ponytail 4 on the other side of the hair band.

11. Join both of these sections with ponytail 8 and secure with a hair elastic.

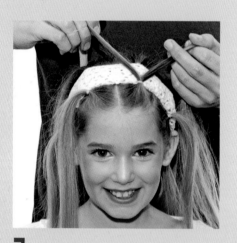

7

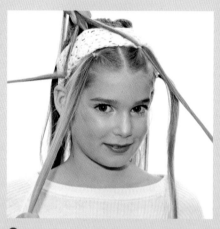

8

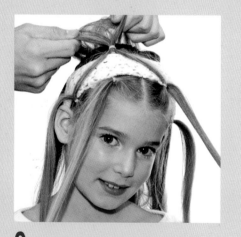

9

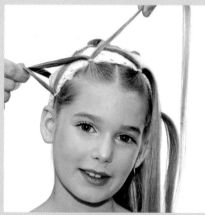

10

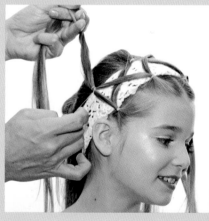

11

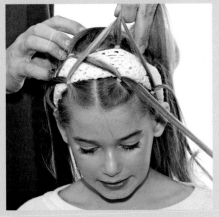

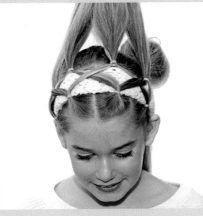

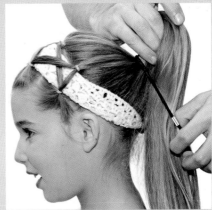

12

13

14

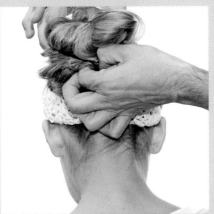

15

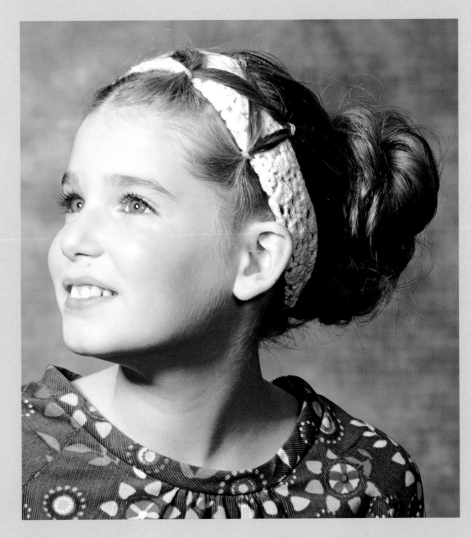

12. Split ponytail 1 into two even sections. Join one of these sections with the loose section of ponytail 3. Join with the hair in ponytail 6 on the other side of the hair band, and secure with a hair elastic.

13. Join the loose sections in ponytails 1 and 2 with ponytail 5. Secure with a hair elastic.

14. Move to the back of the head and gather all of the hair in a high ponytail.

15. Twist the ponytail into a bun and secure with bobby pins. Mist with holding spray.

Wavy Crown

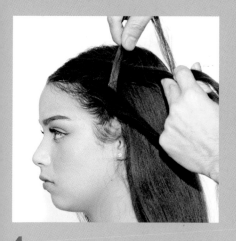

1. Wash and blow dry the hair. Rub moisturizing cream on all the hair to make it smooth. Grasp three small sections of hair at the hairline.

2. Number the sections of hair from 1 to 3, with section 3 closest to the top of the head. Draw section 2 over section 1 and then draw section 1 over section 3. Section 3 will now be at the bottom of the braid.

3. Release section 3 from your grip so that it hangs loose, and grasp a new section of hair from the top of the head. This will replace the section you just released and allow you to continue braiding the hair.

4. Bring the new section at the top of the head under the middle portion, then bring the bottom section upwards under the middle section.

1

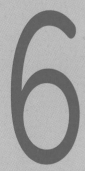

6

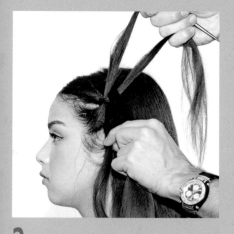

2

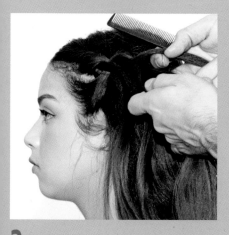

3

4

Have some fun with this wavy masterpiece. Create a hair band of braided hair around the top of the head and then curl the loose ends in a wonderful wave. Fun, playful, and easy!

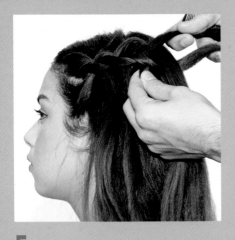

5

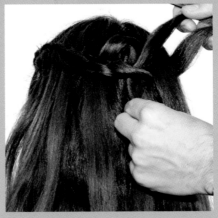

6

5. As in Step 3, release the bottom most section of the braid so that it hangs loose.

6. Grasp a section of hair from above the braid to replace the section that is now loose.

7. Continue in this manner to make a braid that runs all around the head, similar to a garland or crown.

8. When you reach the other side of the head, braid the hair into an ordinary braid and secure it at the end with a hair elastic.

9. Curl the sections of hair that hang loose from the braided crown with a medium curling iron.

10. Work your way around the entire head to curl all these sections of hair.

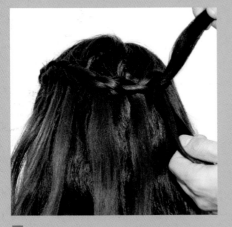

7

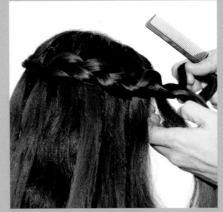

8

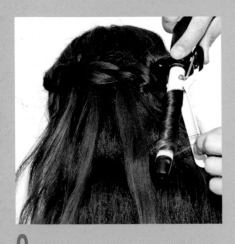

9

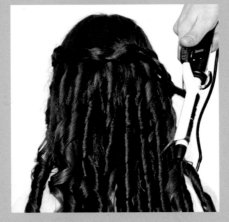

10

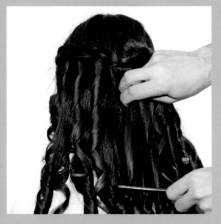

11

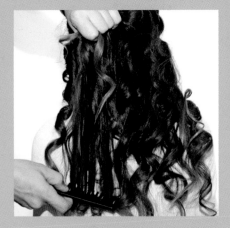

12

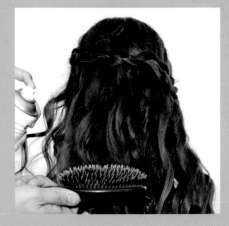

13

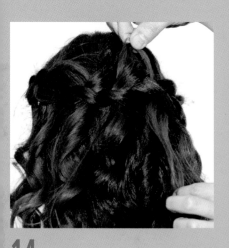

14

11. Gently comb out the curls to soften them.

12. Make sure that you hold the hair under the braid while you brush out the curls so that you don't damage the braid.

13. For a wavier look, mist holding spray onto a bristle brush and then brush out the curls.

14. Thicken the braided crown by gently tugging on the braided sections a little bit.

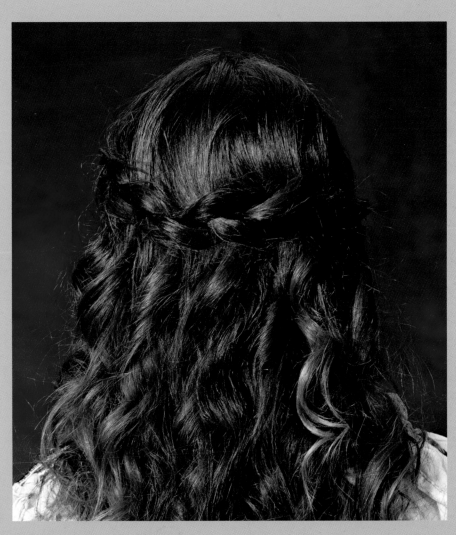

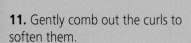

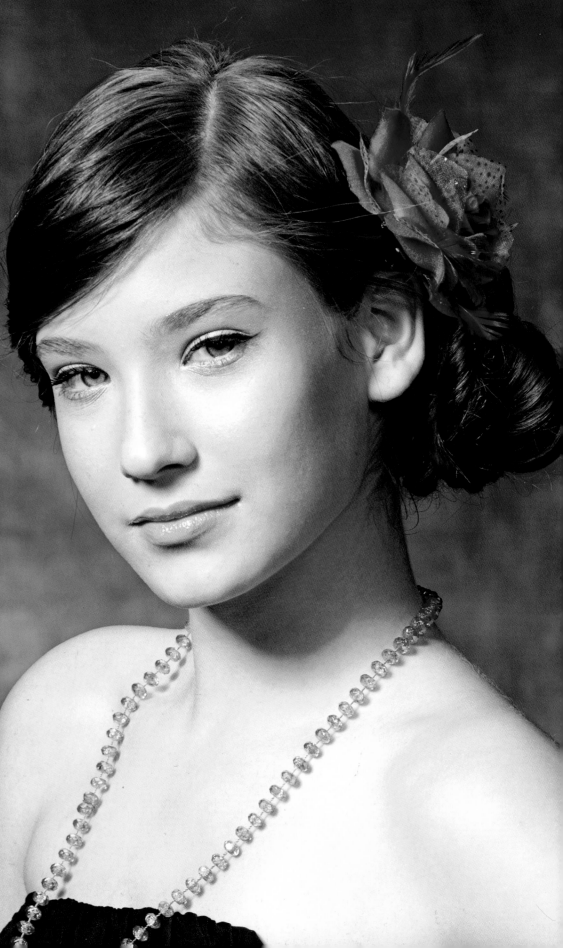

Swirled Sophistication

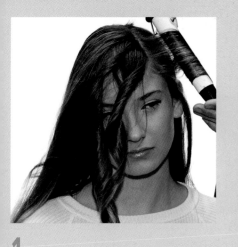

1. Wash and blow dry the hair. Curl small sections of hair with a medium curling iron.

2. Work your way all around the head to curl all of the hair. Mist with holding spray.

3. Separate the hair into two sections with a side part from the brow to the nape of the neck.

4. Divide the hair on the left side of the part into front and back sections. Twist each section around itself and towards the left.

7

1

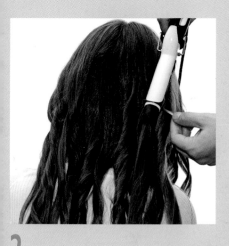

2

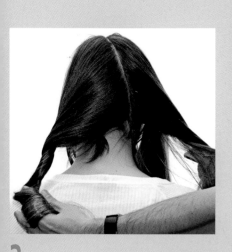

3

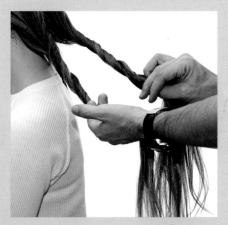

4

Create an elegant impression with this stylish side style. Sleek and fresh, it's also really easy to make.

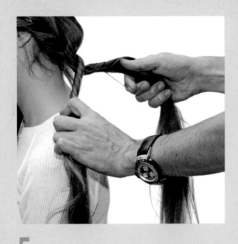

5

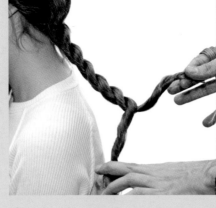

6

5. Twist both twisted sections of hair together, holding them securely so that you don't lose the twist.

6. Continue twisting the twisted sections of hair together until you reach the end of the hair.

7. Fold the twisted hair upwards and then bring it towards the left side of the head.

8. Twist the twisted hair to form a bun and secure it over the ear.

9. Repeat this process on the other side of the head, first dividing the hair into two sections and then twisting each section around itself.

10. When twisting the sections of hair together, make sure you continue to hold the twist in each section.

11. Continue twisting together the twisted sections of hair until you reach the end of the hair.

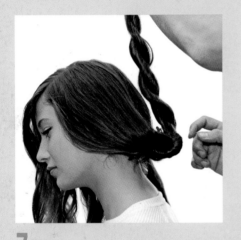

7

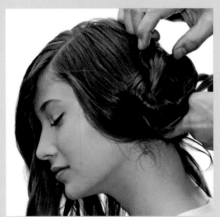

8

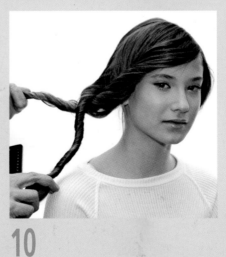

9

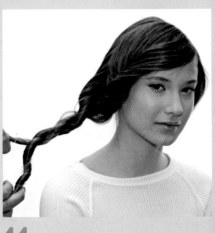

10

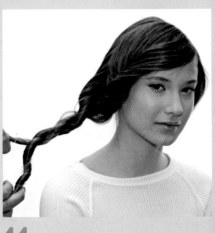

11

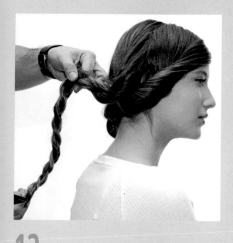

12

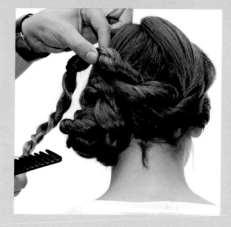

13

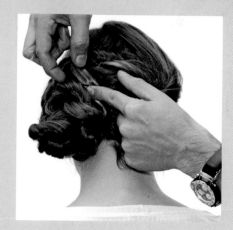

14

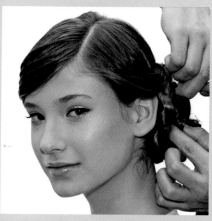

15

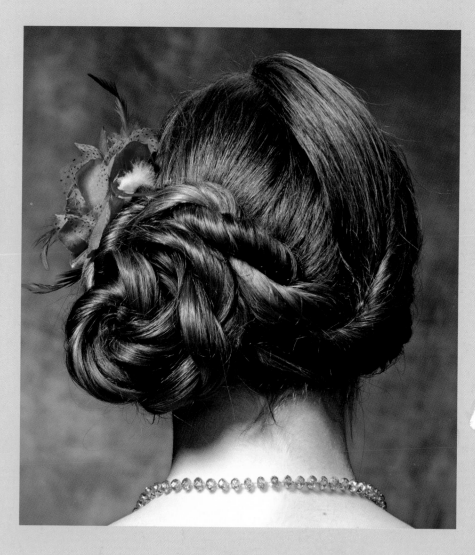

12. Fold the twisted hair upwards and bring it towards the left side of the head.

13. Fold the hair so that it is adjacent to the first twist of hair.

14. Twist the hair around the twisted bun and secure with hair pins.

15. Use as many pins as you need to secure the hair in place. Mist with holding spray.

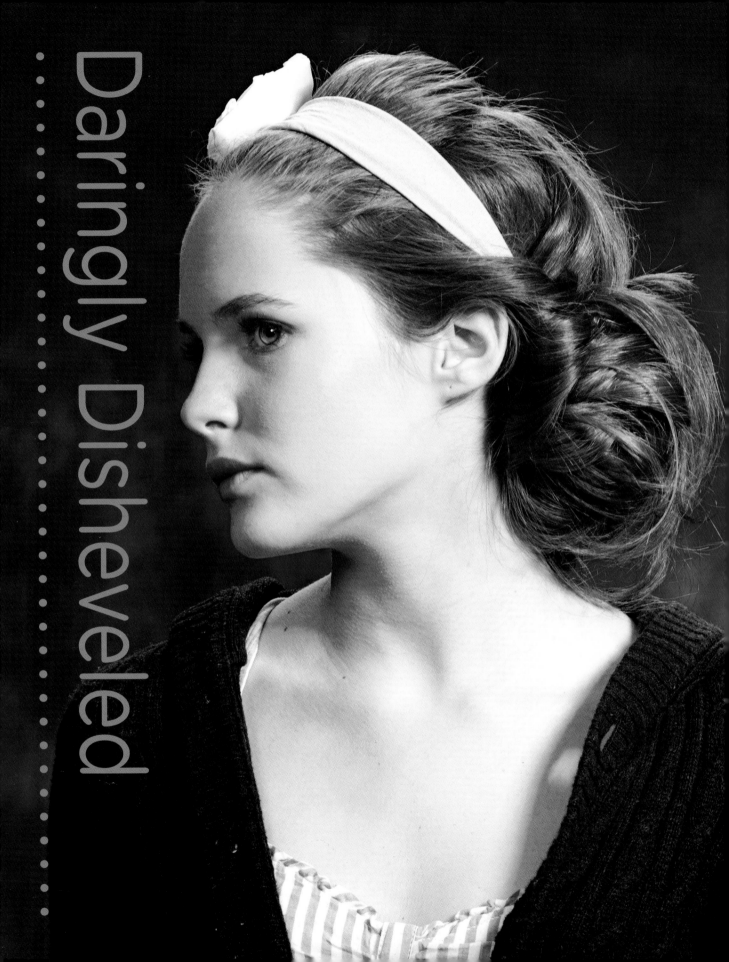

Daringly Disheveled

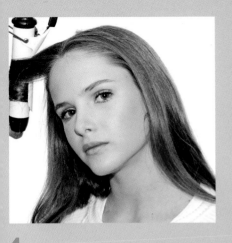

1

1. Wash the hair, rub a bit of mousse into it, and then blow dry it. Curl the hair all around the head into large rolls, using a medium curling iron.

2. Spray the hair with styling spray and wait about five minutes for the spray to dry.

3. Grasp the hair at the front of the brow and mist it at the roots with hair spray.

4. Backcomb the roots to create volume.

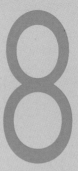

8

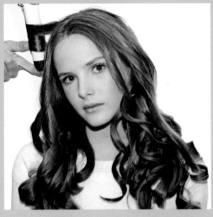

2

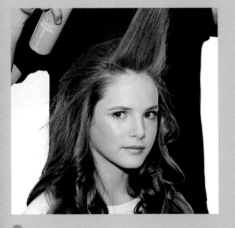

3

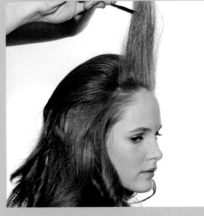

4

While some hairstyles are serenely sleek, others charm by looking spontaneously spunky. This style definitely falls into the latter category!

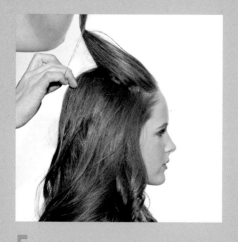

5

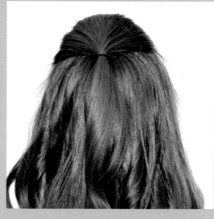

6

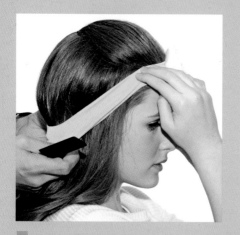

7

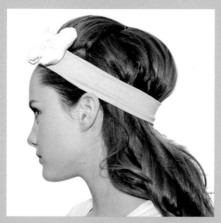

8

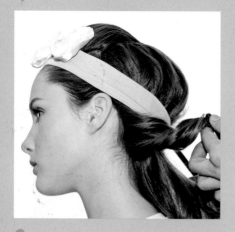

9

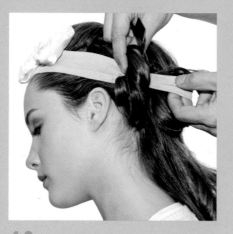

10

5. Mist the hair with a bit of hair spray and then gently brush it out, while drawing it backwards, to create a smooth look. Make sure you don't reduce the volume while brushing it. Secure this section of hair with a hair elastic at the crown of the head.

6. Place the elastic band close to the scalp.

7. Wrap an elastic hair band around the head. Make sure the hair band is tight, as you'll be using it as a base for the hairstyle.

8. Position the hair band so that it lies along the hairline at the front of the head and just above the ear line all around the head. The hair band should lie on top of the hair.

9. Grasp a section of hair extending below the hair band and behind the left ear, and twist it upwards.

10. Pull the hair band here away from the head a bit and tuck the twisted section of hair into it so that the hair conceals this part of the hair band.

11. Move your way towards the nape of the neck, drawing out another section of hair, twisting it upwards and tucking it under the hair band, as you did previously.

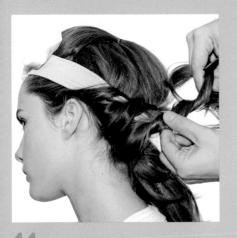

11

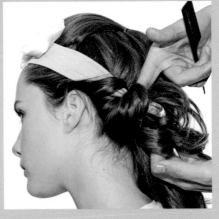

12

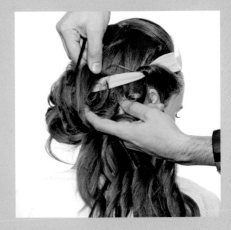

13

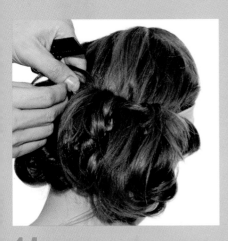

14

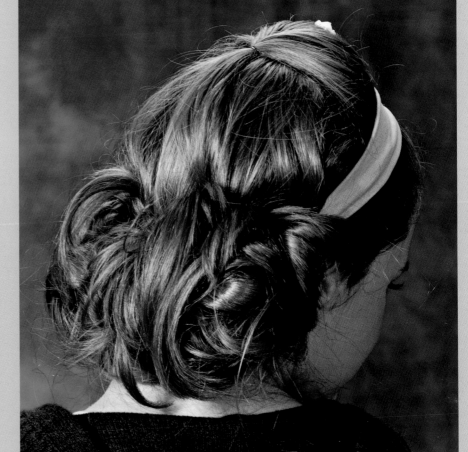

12. If the hair is particularly long, roll it around the hair band twice every time.

13. Continue in this matter all the way around the head, until you reach the right ear. Make sure you conceal the hair band entirely as you wrap it with sections of hair.

14. After wrapping all the hair around the hair band, insert hair pins close to the hair band to secure the wraps. Mist with holding spray.

Maze o' Braids

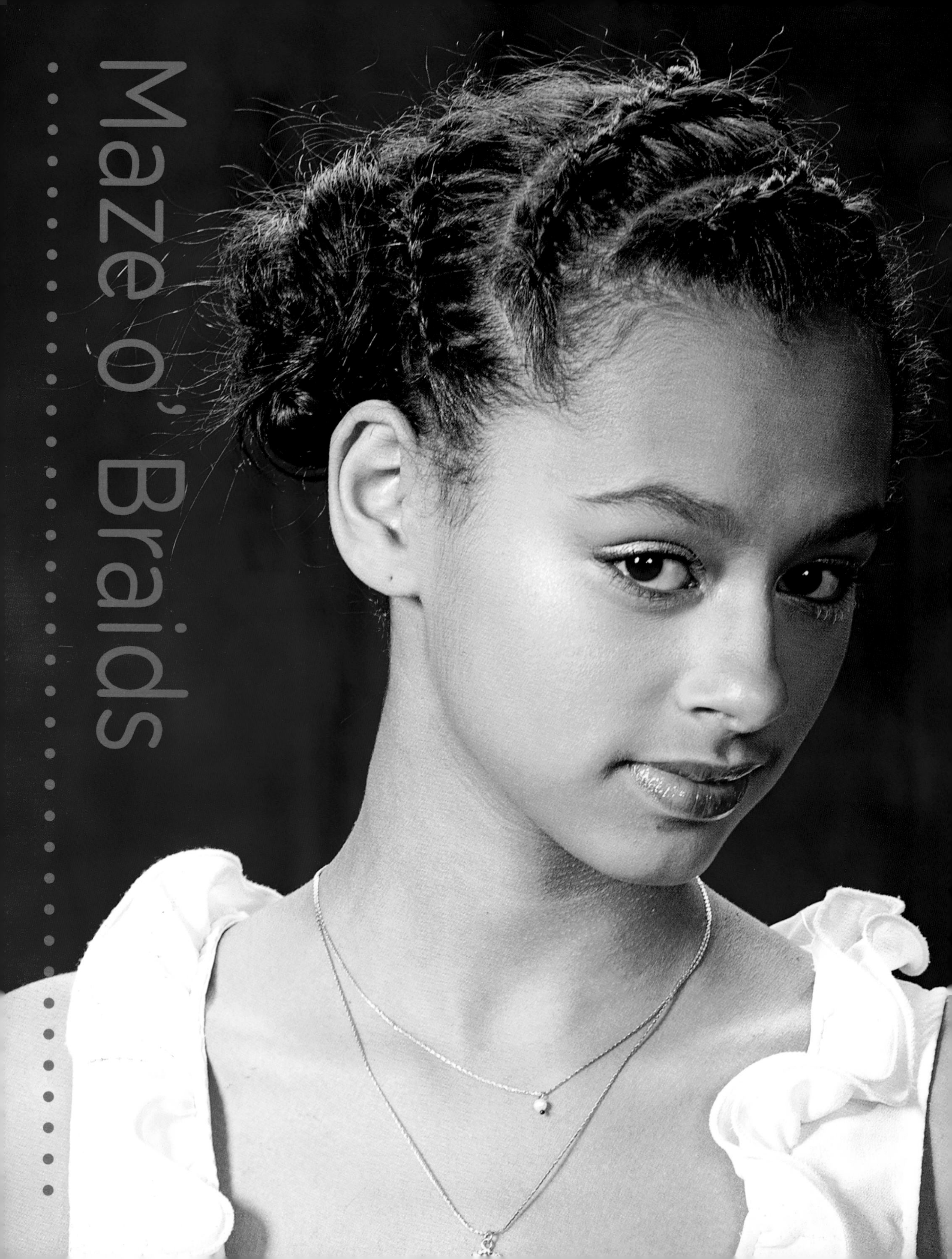

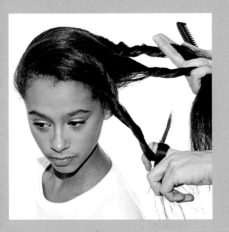

1. Wash and blow dry the hair straight. Divide the hair into four sections: one front section, one back section, and two middle sections. Draw the hair in the first three sections to the left side of the head. Collect the hair in the back section in a ponytail.

2. Draw out a small section of hair from the right corner of the front section, divide it into three sections, and begin making an inside-out French braid. This means you'll be passing the left and right sections of hair under the middle section, rather than over it.

3. Continue braiding the hair towards the left side of the head, adding a bit of hair to each section as you work your way along the braid.

4. Continue weaving the braid towards the front of the head. Make sure the sections are tidy and clearly defined so that the braid really sticks out. This means you'll be weaving the side sections under the middle section, rather than over it.

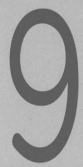

1

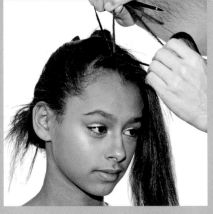

2

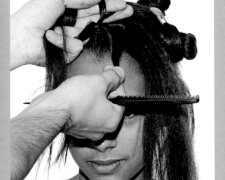

3

4

Put a twist on standard braids (literally!) with this fun design. It's easy to do, but creates an awesomely intricate look.

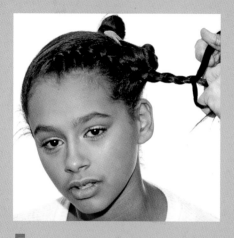

5

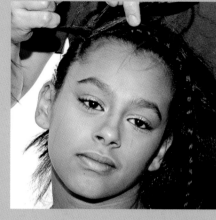
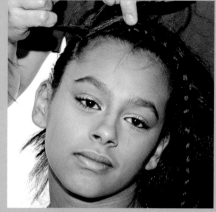

6

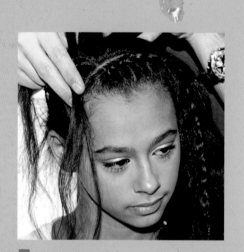

7

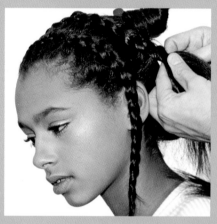

8

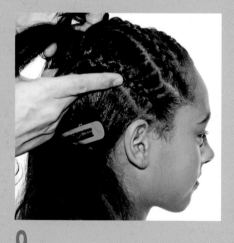

9

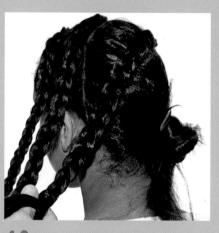

10

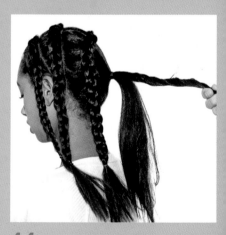

11

5. Continue the braid until you reach the ends of the hair and secure it with a hair elastic.

6. Start making a similar braid in the second section of hair.

7. Make this braid in exactly the same way. Work slowly to make sure that the braid is tight, tidy, and woven close to the scalp.

8. Secure the end of the second braid with a hair elastic.

9. Make a similar braid in the third section of hair.

10. Now you should have three inside-out French braids, all of them beginning on one side of the head and finishing on the other.

11. Move to the hair that's collected in a ponytail at the back of the head. Grasp one-quarter of the ponytail and gently twist it around itself.

12. Grasp a strand of hair from this twisted section and push the rest of the hair towards the scalp to create a twisted pillow of hair. Secure the hair at the base of the ponytail with bobby pins.

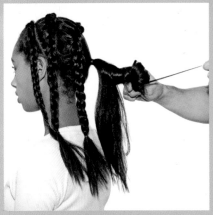

12

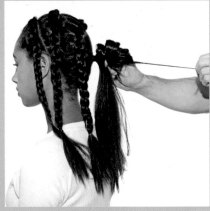

13

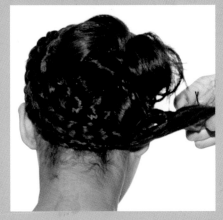

14

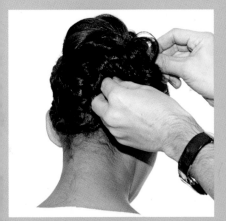

15

13. Repeat this process with the rest of the hair in this ponytail, twisting a quarter section every time and pushing it towards the scalp. At the end, you should have four messy loops secured to the head with bobby pins.

14. Hold the ends of the three braids together and draw them under the collection of loops.

15. Secure the ends of the braids at the base of the ponytail. Mist with holding spray.

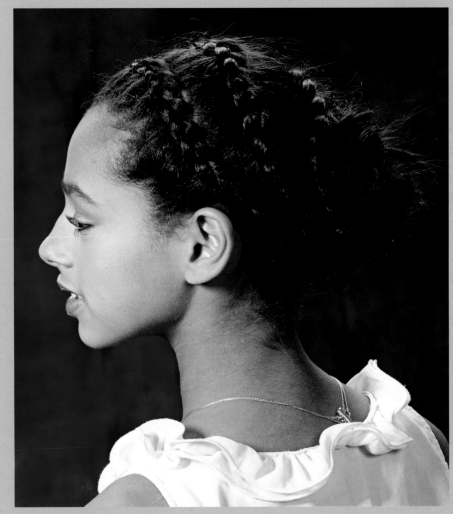

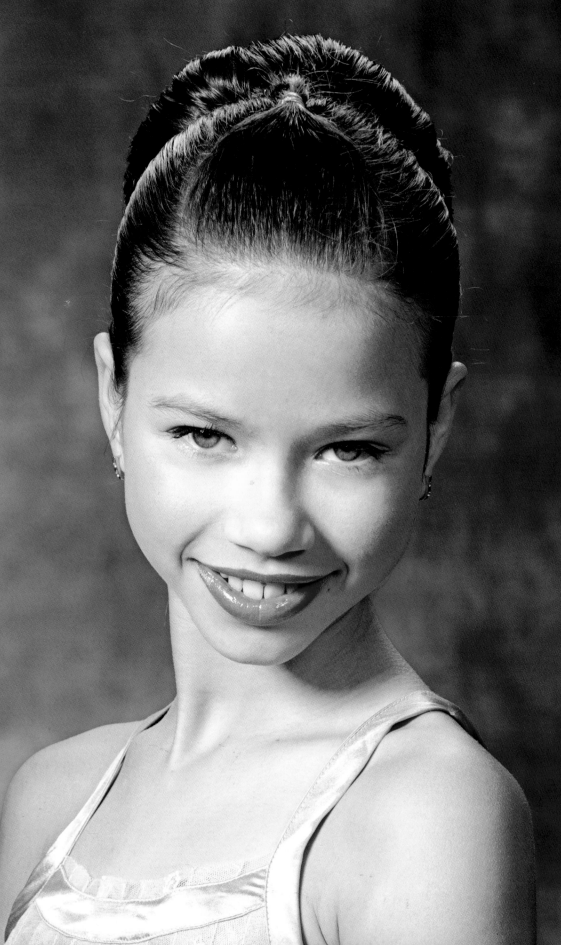

Fantastically Flirty

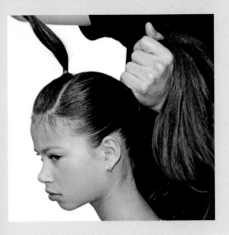

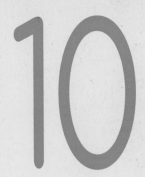

1. Wash and blow dry the hair. Make a triangular part at the front of the head and gather the hair in a ponytail. Gather the rest of the hair at the back of the head in a high ponytail.

2. Mist the hair with hair spray to give it a smooth, clean look.

3. Divide the hair in the triangular ponytail into two even sections. Twist each section around itself so that it looks like a twisted rope of hair.

4. Cross one of the twisted sections over the other and twist them together, rotating them slightly as you twist.

1

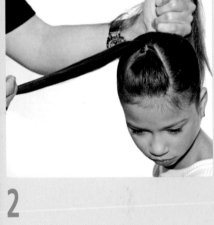
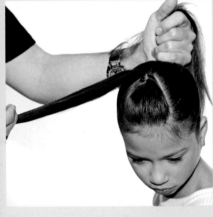

2

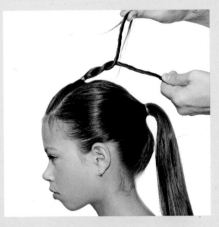

3

4

This hairstyle is as much fun to make as it is to wear. You'll need a 32-inch ribbon— choose something that's bright, thick, and flirty!

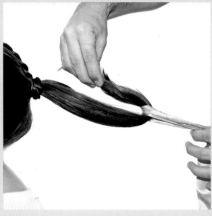

5

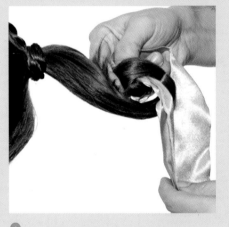

7

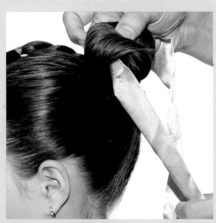

9

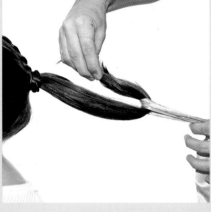

6

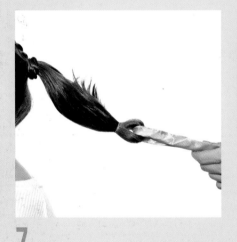

8

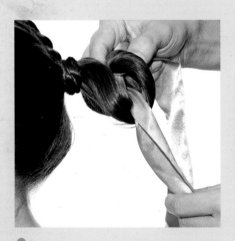

10

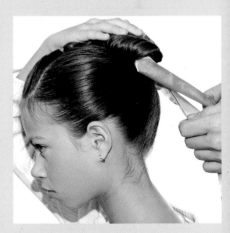

11

5. Continue twisting the sections of hair together until you reach the ends of the hair, and secure with a hair elastic. Wrap the twisted hair around the base of the high ponytail.

6. Fold a 32-inch ribbon in half. Tuck the bottom of the ponytail into the folded ribbon. Draw the ponytail upwards and draw the ends of the ribbon downwards. Make sure the ribbon hangs evenly on either side of the ponytail.

7. Secure the folded ponytail around the ribbon using a hair elastic so that the ribbon is held in a loop at the end of the ponytail.

8. Gently roll the ponytail upwards towards the head. Make sure the ribbon stays securely tucked into the loop.

9. Continue rolling the hair until you reach the scalp.

10. Make sure that the hair is tightly rolled.

11. When the hair is rolled all the way up to the scalp, ask the person whose hair you are styling to hold the

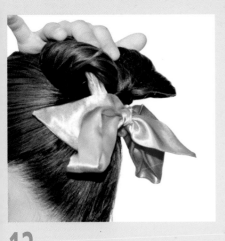

12

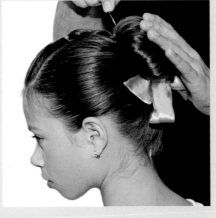

13

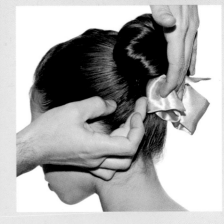

14

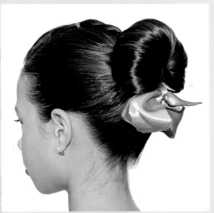

15

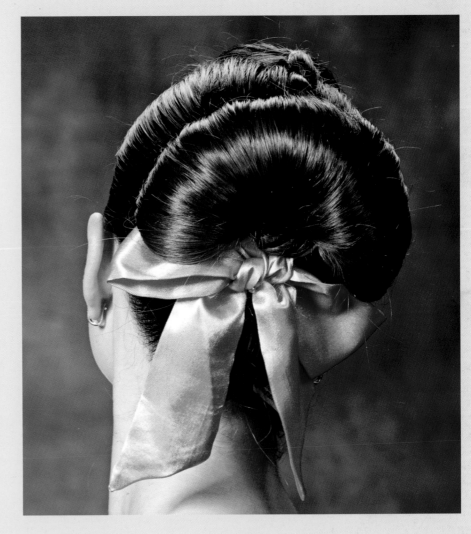

roll in place. Take the ends of the ribbon and tie a secure knot on the underside of the rolled hair.

12. Tie the ends of the knotted ribbon into a bow.

13. Secure the rolled hair to the head with hair pins.

14. Gently open the rolled hair by drawing the hair towards the right and left sides of the head, like a fan. Insert pins along the fan to secure it in place.

15. Mist with holding spray.

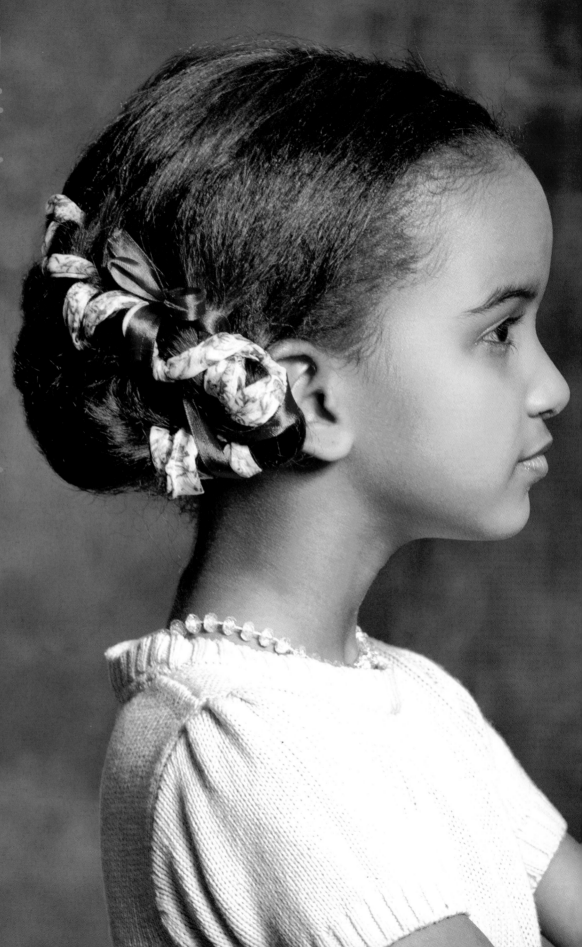

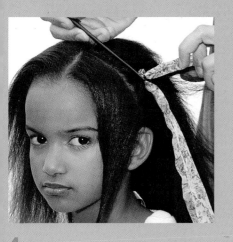

1

1. Wash and blow dry the hair. Make a middle part from the brow to the nape of the neck to divide the hair into two even sections. Fold a 32-inch scarf in half and secure it to a section of hair above and behind the left ear with a hair elastic.

2. Grasp a section of hair at the hairline on the left side of the head, and grasp the two sides of the scarf.

3. Wrap one section of the scarf over the hair.

4. Draw this section of hair over the other side of the scarf.

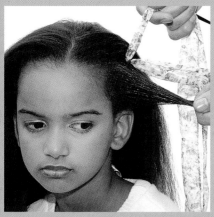

2

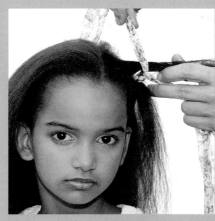

3

4

Here's a fun design that's colorful, too! When choosing the scarf and ribbon, make sure they are both at least 32 inches long. You'll also need a dull plastic needle.

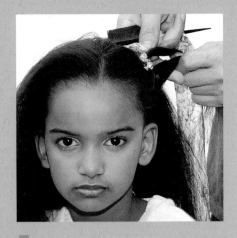

5

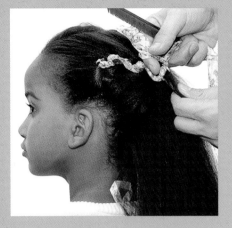

6

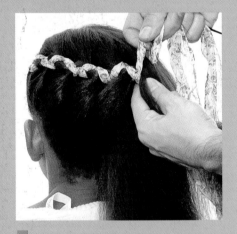

7

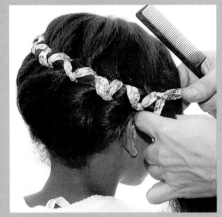

8

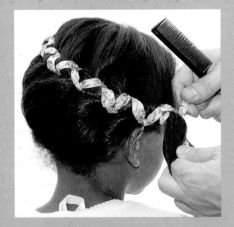

9

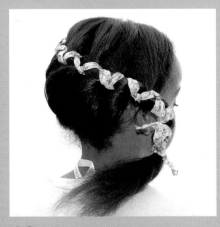

10

5. Draw the scarf around the hair so that the hair section is now located between the two sides of the scarf. Grasp another section of hair from the hairline and join it with the closest side of the scarf.

6. Number the sections from 1 to 3 and start braiding them by drawing section 3 under section 2, and section 1 under section 3. As you proceed, add small sections of hair on either side of the braid.

7. Continue this process, working your way around the back of the head, from the left side towards the right side. Keep the hair relatively high at the back of the head while adding sections of hair to the braid.

8. Continue the braid until you reach the end of the hair.

9. Wrap the ends of the scarf around the end of the hair and tie them in a secure knot.

10. Tie the scarf ends in a tidy bow and mist with holding spray.

11. Thread a dull plastic needle with a 32-inch piece of ribbon. Poke the needle in and out of the hair at the top of the braid to secure it in place. Gently pull one end of the ribbon until the two sides hang evenly. Keep the needle threaded on one side of the ribbon.

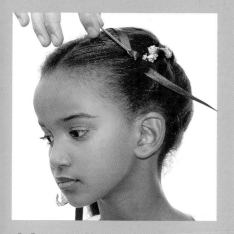
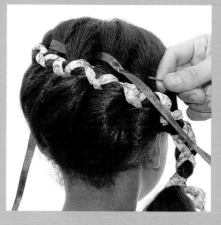
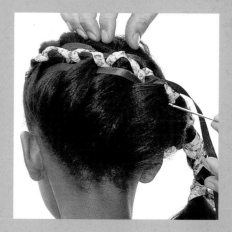

11   **12**   **13**

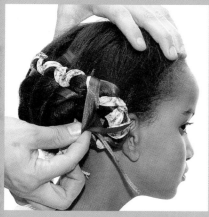

14

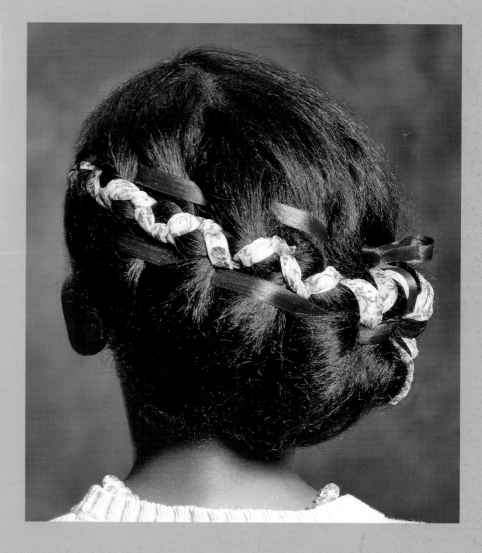

12. Use the needle to weave the ribbon in and out of the hair along the braid. Weave the ribbon so that it contrasts with the scarf in the braid.

13. When you reach the end of the braid, let the ribbon hang loose. Thread the other side of the ribbon with the needle and weave it through the hair on the other side of the braid.

14. Tie the ends of the ribbon in a bow at the end of the braid. Mist with holding spray.

• • • • • • • • • •

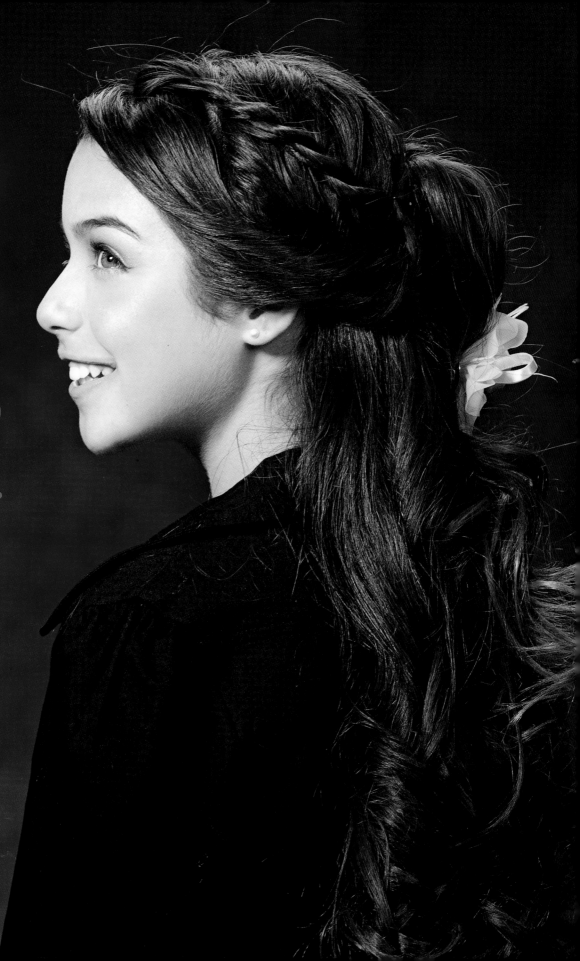

Sugar 'n' Spice

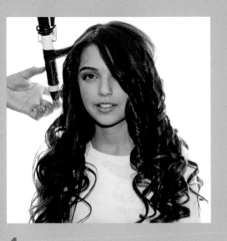

1. Wash and blow dry the hair. Curl the hair with a medium curling iron to create a wavy look.

2. Draw aside a 1-inch section of hair from just behind the bangs and divide it into two equal sections.

3. Twist each section around itself and then cross the two twisted sections to form an X.

4. Continue twisting these sections of hair together. Every time you twist, integrate a bit of hair from above the twisted sections into the bottom section of the X.

12

1

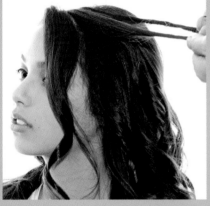

2

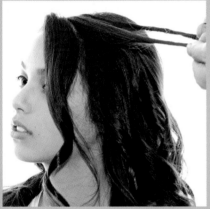

3

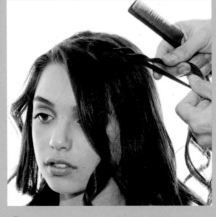

4

This masterpiece hairstyle has a bit of everything that's nice! It's got braids, curls, twirls, and a fun floral hair pin.

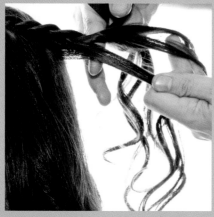

5

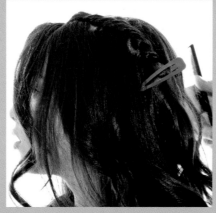

6

5. At every stage, you'll add a small section of hair from above the twist, passing it under the twisted rope.

6. When the twisted rope reaches the back of the head, secure with a hair clip and let the ends hang loose.

7. Repeat this process on the other side of the head.

8. Divide the bangs with a side part. Draw the bangs on the left side of the part backwards, while twisting them inwards. When they reach the back of the head, join them with the twisted rope of hair and secure with a hair elastic.

9. Fold the hair upwards and secure with bobby pins inserted in an X-shape.

10. Roll the ends of hair in this section so that they cover the pins holding the hair in place, and pin the roll with bobby pins.

11. Draw the bangs on the right side of the part backwards. Twist them inwards and then join them with the twisted rope of hair on this side of the head. Fold the hair upwards and secure with bobby pins.

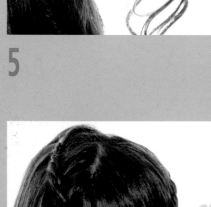

7

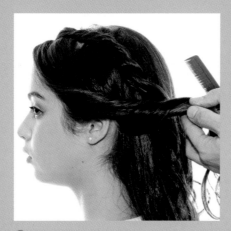

8

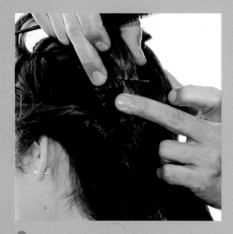

9

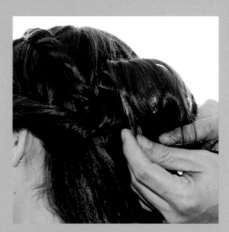

10

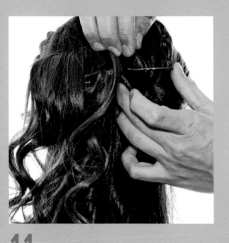

11

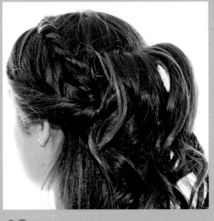

12

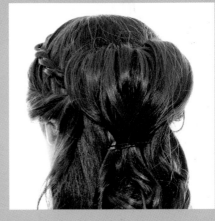

13

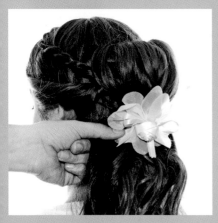

14

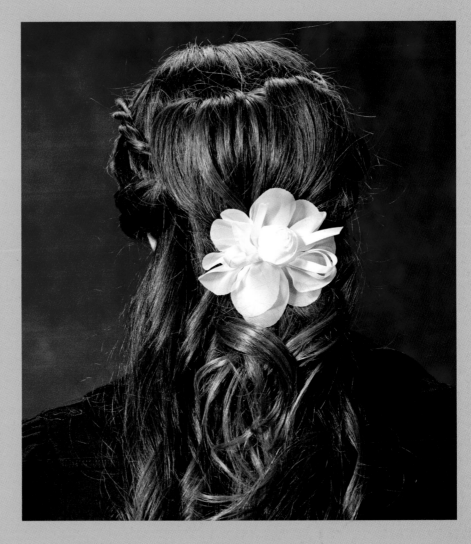

12. Roll the ends of hair in this section as you did in Step 10 and secure with bobby pins.

13. Draw all the loose hair together at the back of the head, about 2½ inches below the waves of hair, and secure with a hair elastic.

14. Add a hair accessory at the back of the hair to conceal the X of hair clips.

 ● ● ● ● ● ● ● ● ●

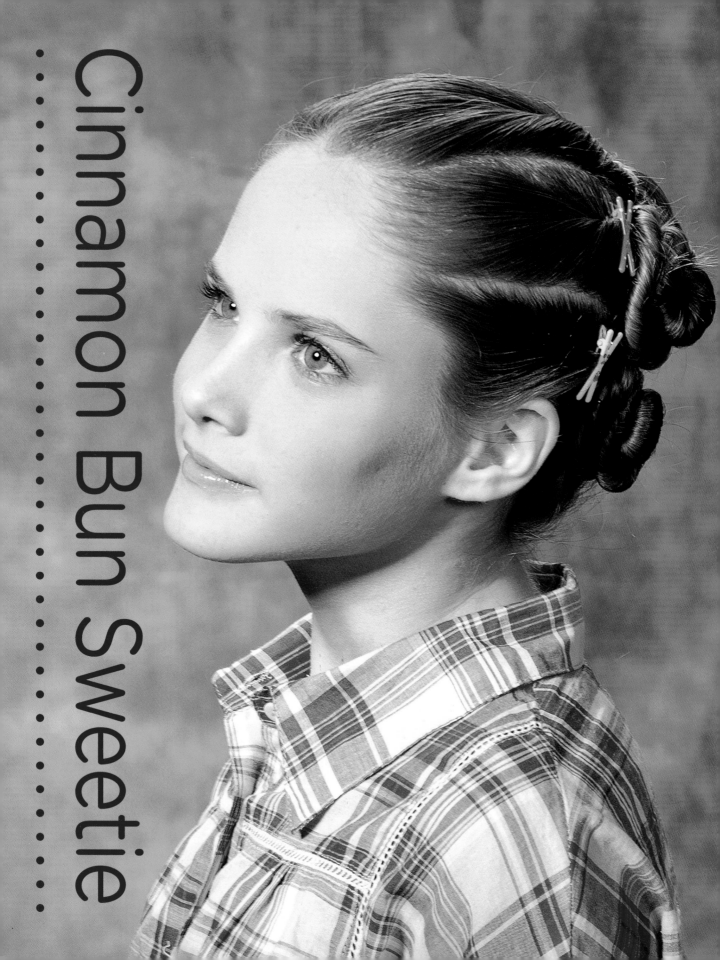

Cinnamon Bun Sweetie

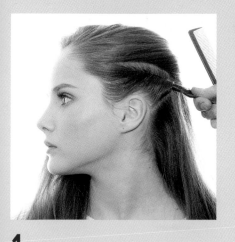

1

1. Wash and blow dry the hair. Gather a section of hair immediately above the left ear that extends from the hairline to just behind the ear. Twist all of this hair tightly inwards, keeping the twist close to the scalp. Keep in mind that you'll be dividing the hair into five sections like this.

2. Draw another section of hair, this one just below the ear, and twist it tightly inwards. Join it with the twist you started in Step 1.

3. Twist the two sections of hair together and then secure with a hair elastic close to the scalp.

4. Draw a section of hair beside the section that you twisted in Step 1. This section should start at the brow and extend just above the ear. Twist this section of hair inwards, keeping it close to the scalp.

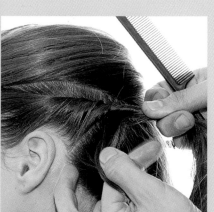

2

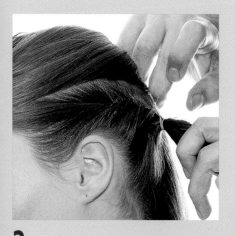

3

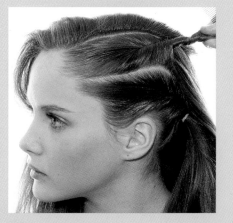

4

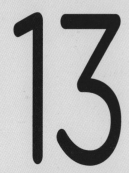

This cute quintet of twirls resembles a super serving of cinnamon buns— and is just as sweet! It's a fabulous and fun way of giving straight hair a bit of a twirl.

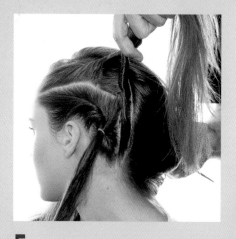

5

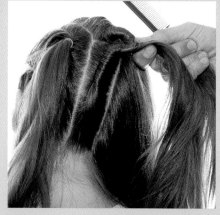

6

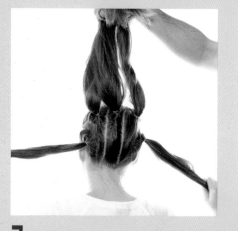

7

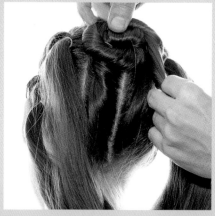

8

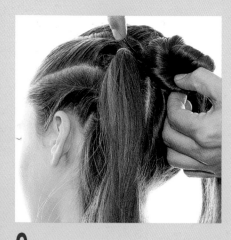

9

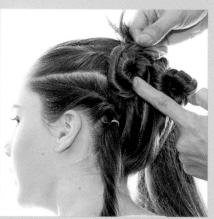

10

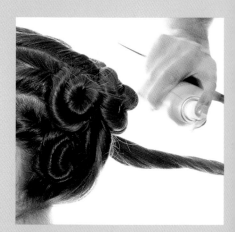

11

5. Grasp a section of hair immediately below this one, starting at the nape of the neck. Twist the hair upwards, joining it with the twist above. Secure both sections of hair with a hair elastic close to the scalp.

6. Continue in this manner all around the head, connecting twists from the top with twists from the bottom.

7. At the end, you should have five ponytails on the head, each one framed by a twist on either side.

8. Hold the middle ponytail, twist it around itself, and then curl the twisted hair into a snail-like shape. Mist the hair with hair spray to hold the twist.

9. Secure the twisted hair in place by pinning the end of the twist to the hair elastic that's holding the ponytail.

10. Repeat this process with the other four ponytails to create a total of five snail-like twists.

11. Mist each swirl of hair with hair spray, both while you're twisting it and afterwards, to make the hairstyle smooth and secure.

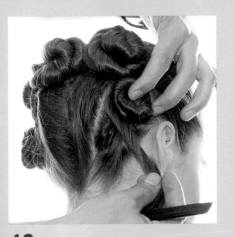

12

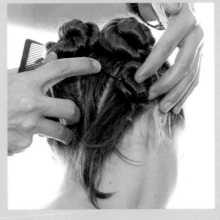

13

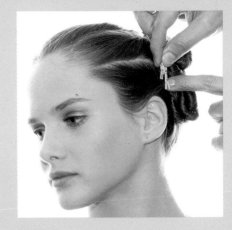

14

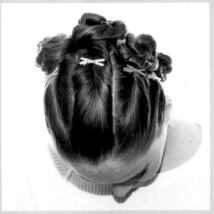

15

12. Twist each section of hair in the same direction when you twist it around itself and when you curl it into the snail-like shape.

13. When securing each twisted section of hair, consider how all five look at the back of the head.

14. If you like, decorate each section of twisted hair with funky barrettes or accessories.

15. Mist with holding spray.

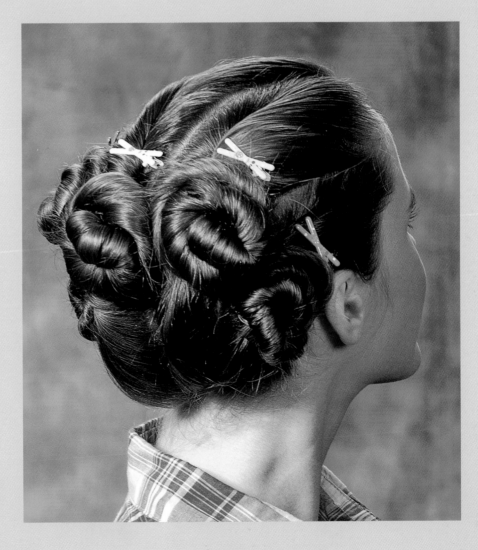

Diamond Darling

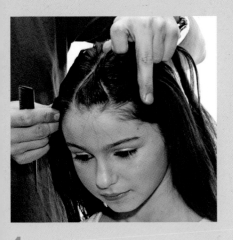

1

1. Wash and blow dry the hair. Rub moisturizing cream on all the hair, then mark off a triangular section at the crown of the head.

2. Secure this hair with a brightly colored hair elastic in a ponytail close to the scalp. This will be the center of the hairstyle, so make sure the ponytail is in the right place and that the hair elastic looks tidy.

3. Gather another section of hair to one side of the middle section and a little farther back. Secure it with a brightly colored hair elastic in a ponytail close to the scalp.

4. Repeat this process on the other side of the middle section. Make sure that the sections are symmetrical and the hair elastics are close to the scalp.

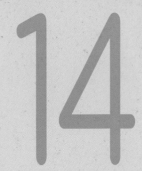

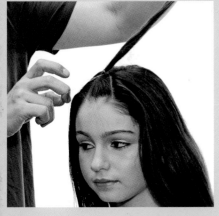

2

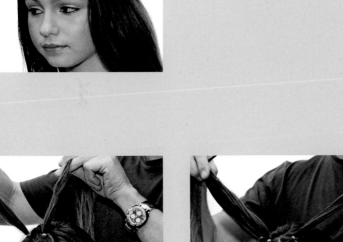

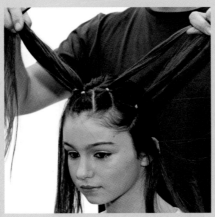

3

4

All you need to create this geometric style is a handful of colorful hair elastics. Make sure the hair is totally tangle-free before you start!

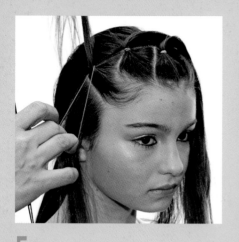

5

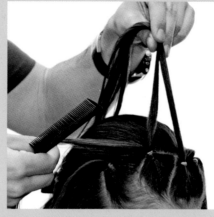

6

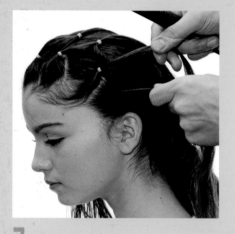

7

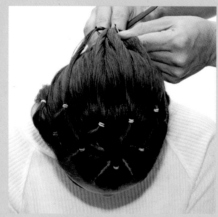

8

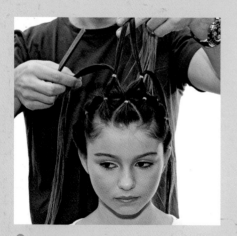

9

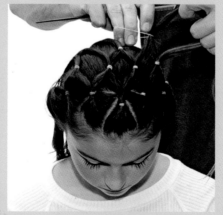

10

5. Repeat this process on either side of the ponytails you've just made to create five ponytails that are similar in size and adjacent to each other.

6. To make the next row of ponytails, divide every ponytail in this first row into two even sections.

7. Make the next row of ponytails by joining adjacent halves of the ponytails. When you come to the ponytails on the left and right sides of the row, use the entire ponytail.

8. Repeat this process to make a second row of ponytails.

9. Now you have triangles of ponytails along the top of the head.

10. Repeat this process to divide the ponytails in the second row into two even sections. Join adjacent sections of these ponytails to make a third row of ponytails.

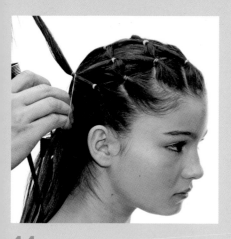

11

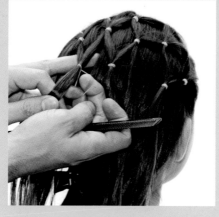

12

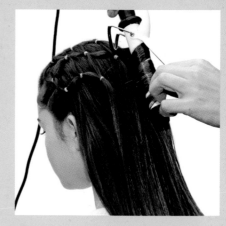

13

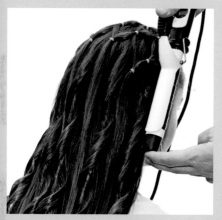

14

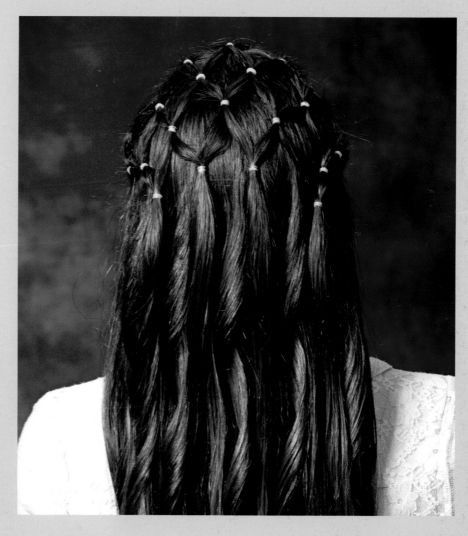

11. Rub each section with moisturizing cream, if necessary, for a smooth, clean look.

12. Now you have a series of diamonds on the top part of the hair.

13. Curl the hair extending from the bottom row of ponytails with a curling iron.

14. Add even more waves by curling the loose hair between each ponytail. Mist with holding spray.

Wonder Weave

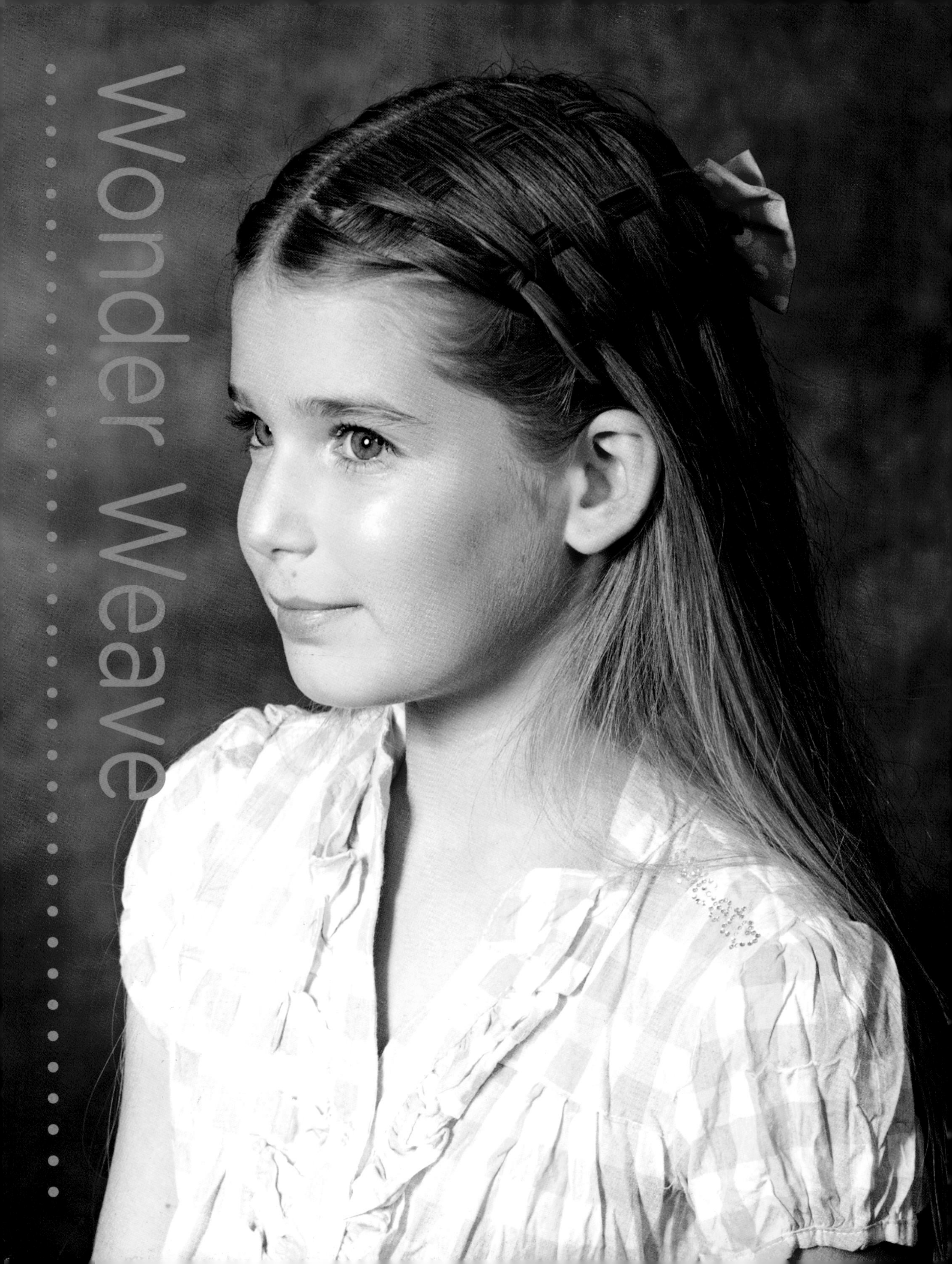

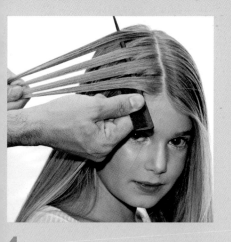

1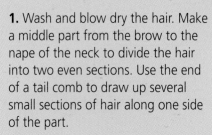

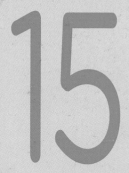

1. Wash and blow dry the hair. Make a middle part from the brow to the nape of the neck to divide the hair into two even sections. Use the end of a tail comb to draw up several small sections of hair along one side of the part.

2. Brush the hair below the lifted sections and mist with holding spray. Continue holding these sections of hair away from the rest of the hair, and draw out a small section of hair at the hairline.

3. Bring the hair from the hairline backwards and under the sections of hair you lifted in Step 1. Secure the hair with a small clip.

4. Bring down the sections of hair that were lifted in Step 1 and lift up the sections that were left down. Draw out another section of hair from the hairline and bring it backwards under these lifted sections.

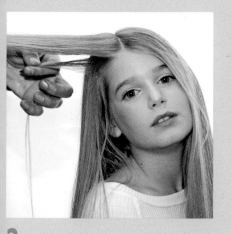

2

Make the most of straight hair by using it to create an elegant weave at the top of the head. Secure the weave with a pretty bow and you're ready for any occasion.

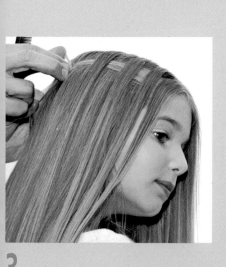

3

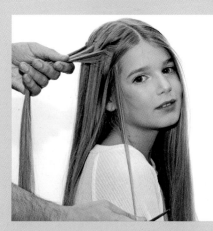

4

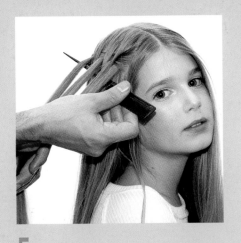

5

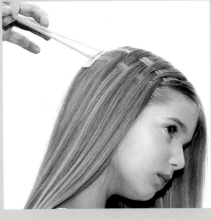

6

5. Repeat the technique in Steps 1 and 2 to weave back another section of hair.

6. Pin this section of hair at the back of the head.

7. Repeat the technique you used in Step 4.

8. As before, weave a small section of hair from the hairline under the lifted sections.

9. Make sure that each section of hair is neatly woven, as this is what allows the pattern to be seen.

10. Secure the woven sections of hair at the back of the head.

11. Repeat this entire process on the other side of the head, drawing back sections of hair at the hairline, weaving them through lifted sections of hair from the part, and pinning them at the back of the head.

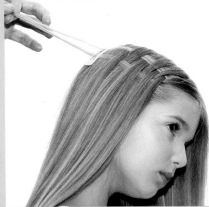

7

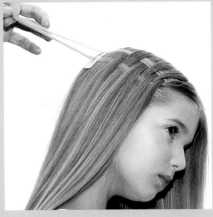

8

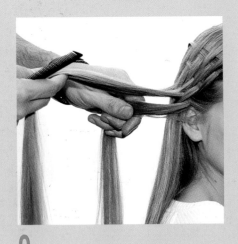

9

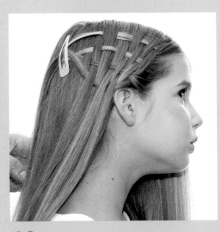

10

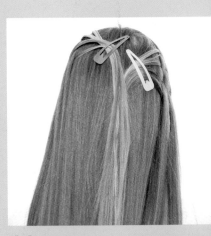

11

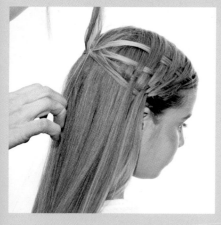

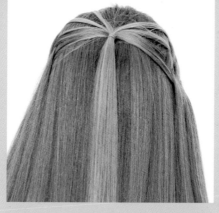

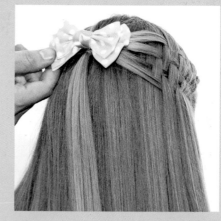

12

13

14

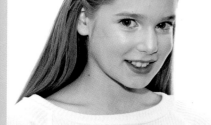

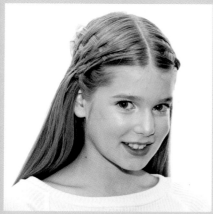

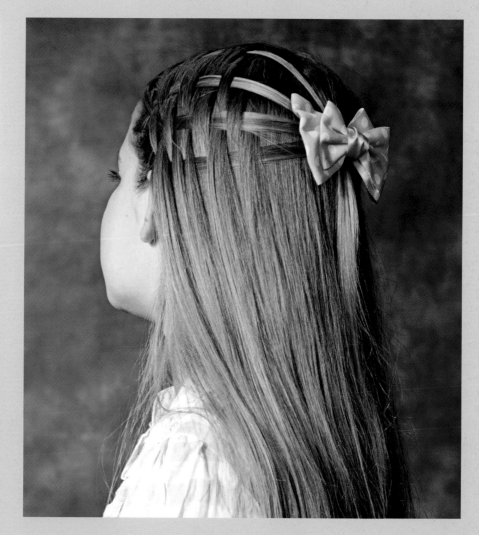

15

12. Gather the sections of hair that you've woven backwards and secure them at the back with a hair elastic.

13. Use a colored hair elastic if you want it to be visible.

14. Add a pretty bow if you like.

15. Mist with holding spray.

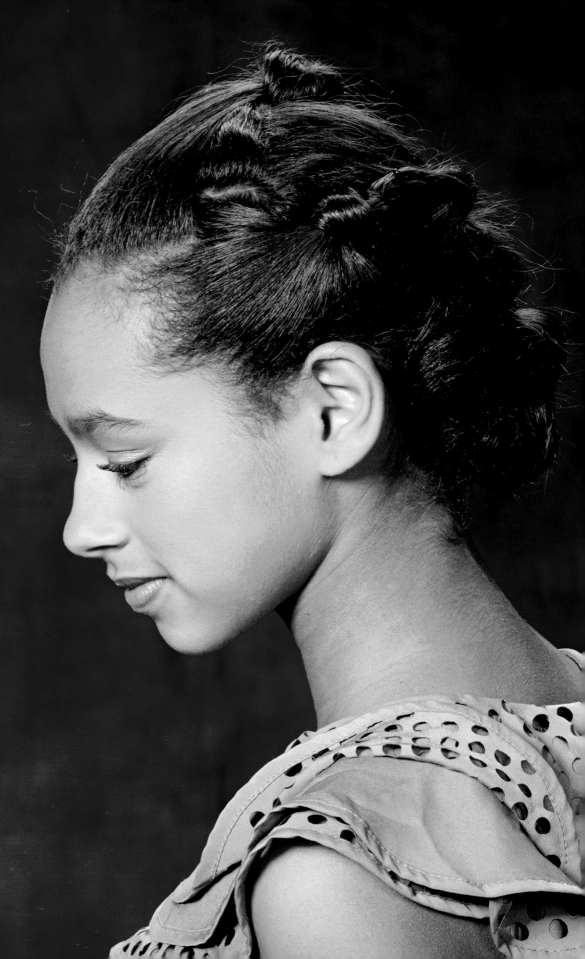

Knotty & Nice

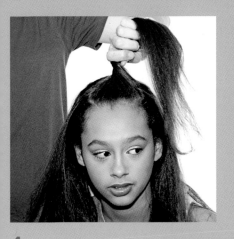

1. Wash and blow dry the hair straight. Gather a square section of hair above the middle of the brow.

2. Twist this section of hair around your fingers to make a loop.

3. Pull the ends of the hair through the loop.

4. Pull the ends gently to create a simple knot.

16

1

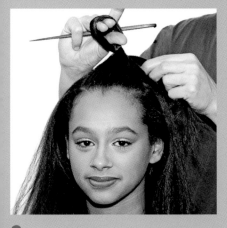

2

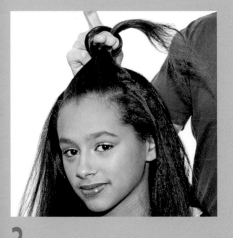

3

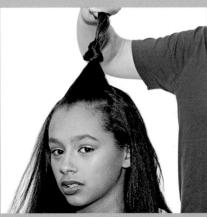

4

Here's a pretty triangular design, made from several knotted sections of hair. It's simple to do, but really impressive. Dress it up with colorful accessories if you like.

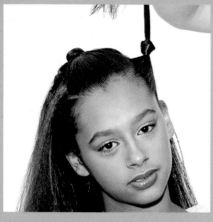

5

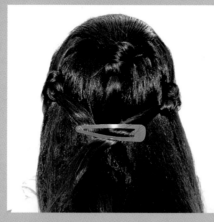

6

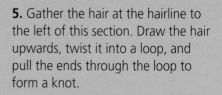

5. Gather the hair at the hairline to the left of this section. Draw the hair upwards, twist it into a loop, and pull the ends through the loop to form a knot.

6. Repeat Step 5 on the other side of the head to form a third knot. Gather the ends of all three knots at the back of the head and secure with a clip.

7. Gather a section of hair on the left side of the head, below the first section, and tie it in a knot. Repeat this process on the other side of the head. Bring the hair extending from both knots over the middle back of the head and tie them together in a knot.

8. Add sections of hair to each section extending from this knot, making the sections longer and thicker. Tie these two sections together to make a knot at the back of the head.

9. Add another section of hair to each of the sections extending from the knot and tie the sections in another knot.

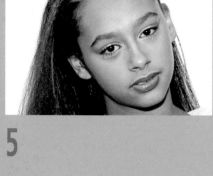

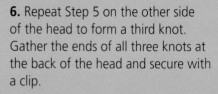

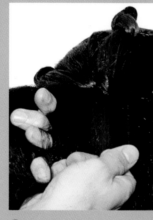

7

8

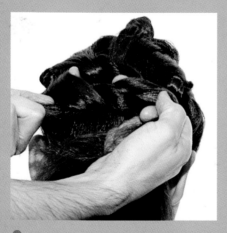

9

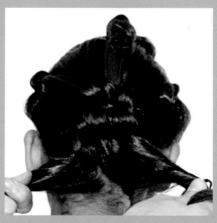

10

11

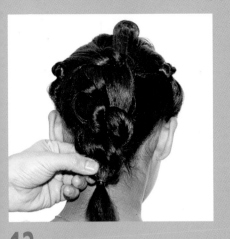

12

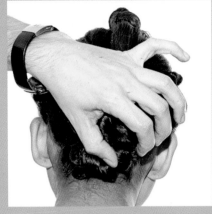

13

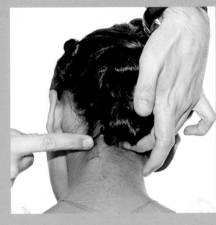

14

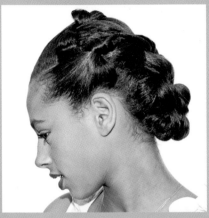

15

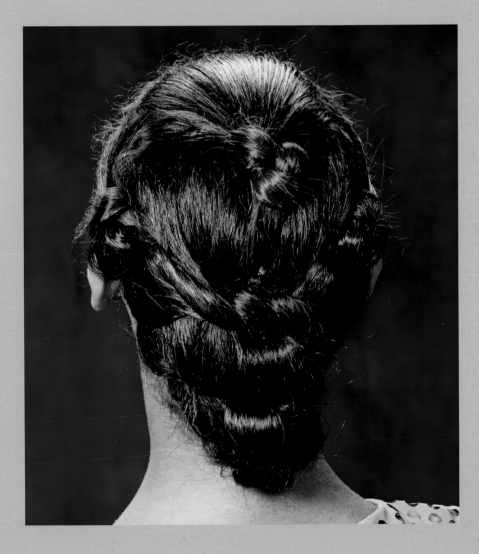

10. Continue knotting the hair in this manner at the back of the head.

11. When you reach the nape of the neck, tie the two sections of hair in a knot.

12. Secure the hair after the last knot with a hair elastic.

13. Tuck the ends of hair after the elastic under the last knot.

14. Hold these ends in place with bobby pins.

15. Mist with holding spray.

Sweetest Surprise

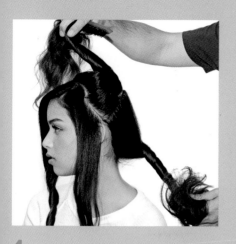

1

1. Wash and blow dry the hair. Divide the hair into two sections with a part from ear to ear over the crown of the head. Divide the hair at the back of the head into an upper and lower section.

2. Gather the hair at the crown of the head in a ponytail and secure with a hair elastic close to the scalp.

3. Use the end of a tail comb to draw out the hair in the ponytail a bit, creating volume.

4. Brush a small section of the hair in this ponytail (about one-fifth of it) upwards and towards the front of the head.

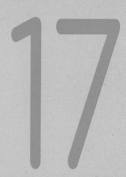

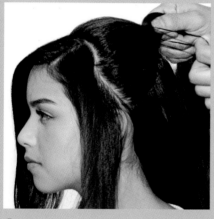

17

2

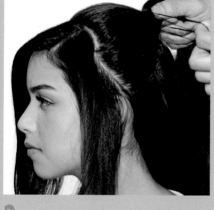

3

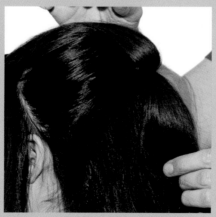

4

Create a natural bow by curling the hair and then wrapping it just so! Like a birthday present waiting to be opened, it's a great design for a Sweet Sixteen or prom.

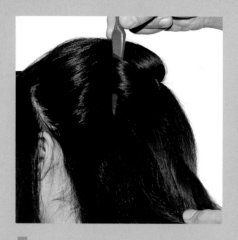

5

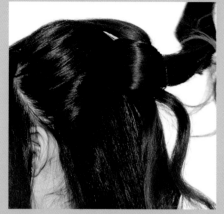

6

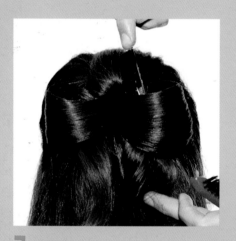

7

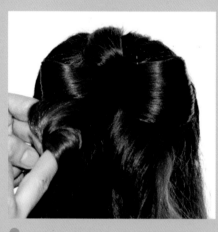

8

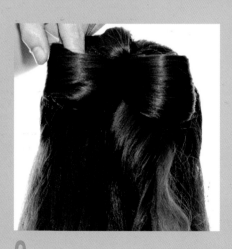

9

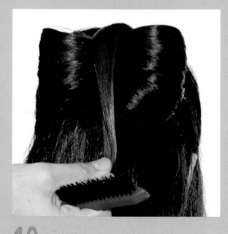

10

5. Divide the rest of the hair in the ponytail into two even sections. Draw the left-most section towards the left and roll it gently towards the right side to make a loop. Secure the loop with bobby pins and allow the ends to hang loose.

6. Repeat this technique on the right side of the ponytail, rolling the hair in the other direction and securing the loop with bobby pins.

7. Insert pins vertically into the loops to make sure they are secure.

8. Wrap the loose hair extending from one of the loops around your finger to form a tight roll.

9. Insert this roll into the loop and secure it with bobby pins. Repeat with the other loop.

10. Draw back the small section of hair that you brushed forward in Step 4.

11. Secure this section of hair at the base of the two loops with bobby pins. Arrange the hair so that it conceals the hair elastic securing the ponytail and completes the bow shape.

12. Place a decorative hair band over the top of the head. Divide the hair in front of the hair band into two sections with a side part. Draw the hair on each side of the part to the back of the head and secure with a hair elastic.

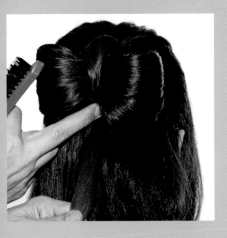

11

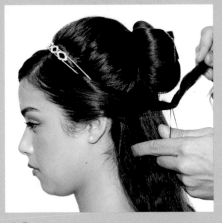

12

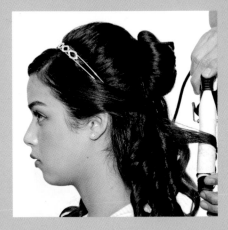

13

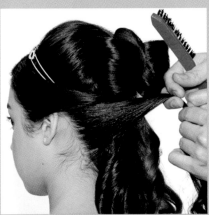

14

13. Curl the loose hair with a curling iron.

14. Gather sections of hair from behind each ear and draw them together at the back of the head. Secure with a hair elastic below the bow. Add more bobby pins, as necessary, to secure all of the hair. Mist with holding spray.

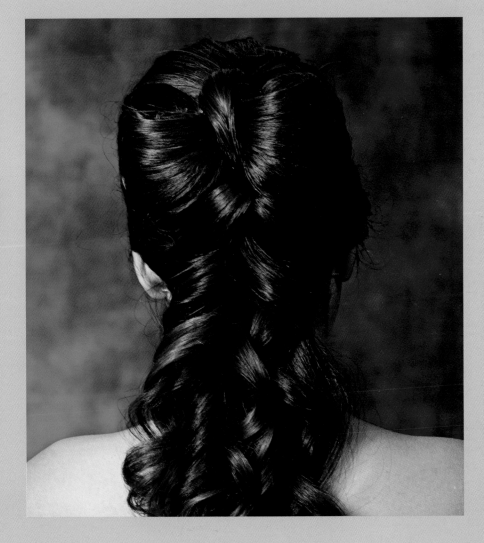

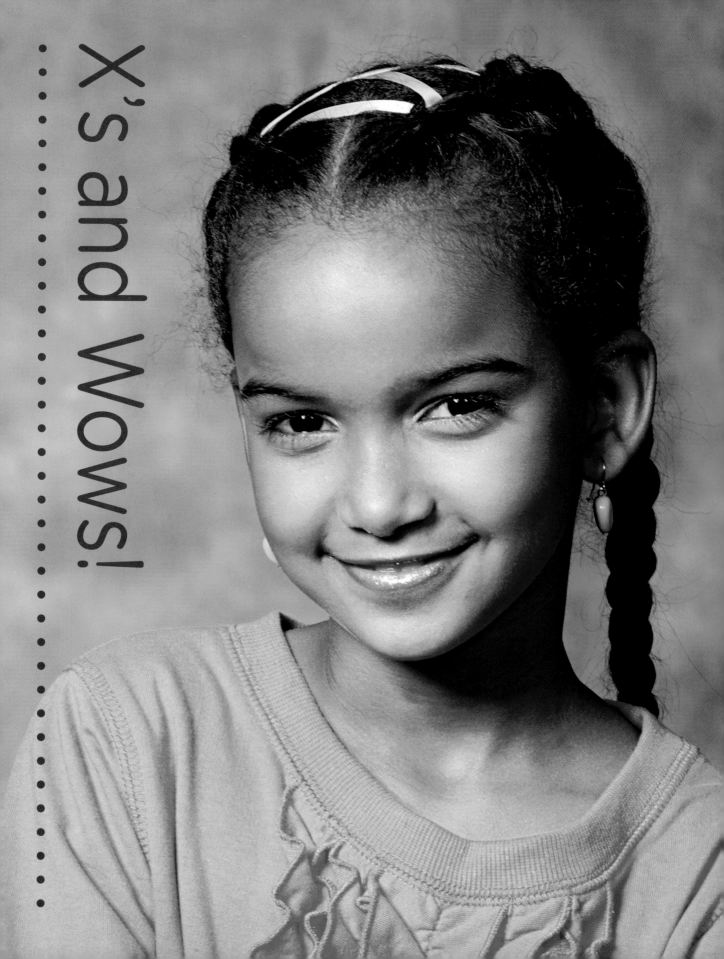

X's and Wows!

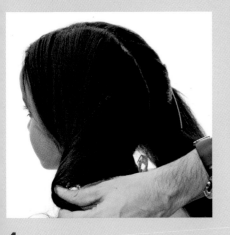

1. Wash and blow dry the hair straight. Make a middle part from the brow to the nape of the neck to divide the hair into two even sections.

2. Hold the hair on the right side of the part with a clip. Grasp a small section of hair on the left side of the part at the hairline and divide it into three equal sections.

3. Number the sections 1 to 3, with section 3 closest to the ear.

4. Bring section 3 under section 2, and then bring section 1 under section 3 to start making the braid.

5. Add a small section of hair to the section that's now closest to the ear, and bring it under the middle section. Add a small section of hair to the section that's farthest from the ear, and then bring it under the new middle section. (See photo page 78)

6. Brush the sections of hair as you work your way along the braid to keep them smooth. Mist with holding spray if necessary. (See photo page 78)

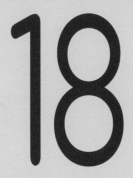

18

Here's a simple hairstyle made fancy thanks to the addition of two bright 32-inch ribbons. You'll also need a dull plastic needle for weaving the ribbons, and a pair of scissors to trim the ribbons at the end.

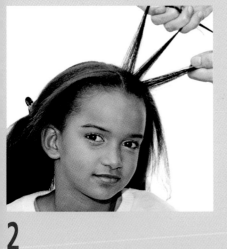

1

2

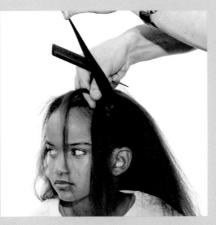

3

4

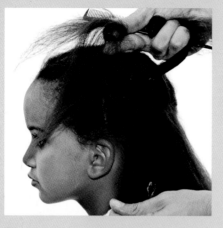

5

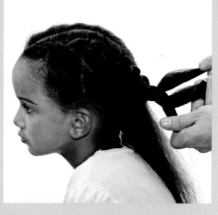

6

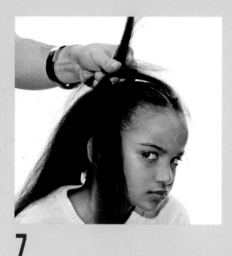

7

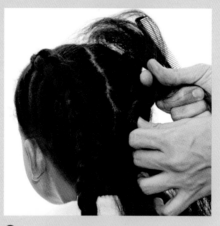

8

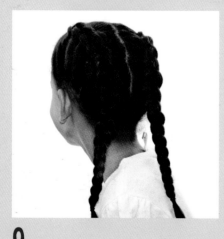

9

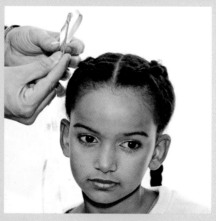

10

7. Continue braiding until you reach the ends of the hair. When you've run out of hair to integrate into the sections, finish by weaving a regular braid and then secure the braid with a hair elastic. Repeat this process on the other side of the part.

8. Continue braiding the hair like this, adding small sections of hair as you work your way along.

9. Secure the end of the braid with a hair elastic.

10. Thread a dull plastic needle with a 32-inch ribbon.

11. Poke the needle in and out of the hair at the top of one braid to secure the ribbon in place. Gently pull the ribbon until both sides are even.

12. Draw one end of the ribbon across the crown of the head and then secure it at the top of the other braid. Draw this end of the ribbon on a diagonal towards the middle of the first braid, and then weave it in and out of the braid to secure it.

13. Continue in this manner, weaving the ribbon back and forth, until you reach the nape of the neck. Repeat

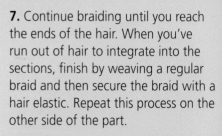

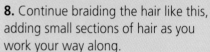

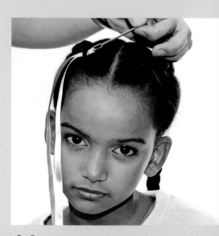

11

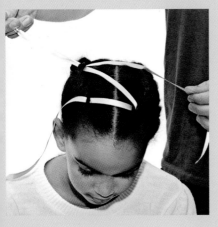

12

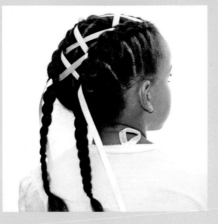

13

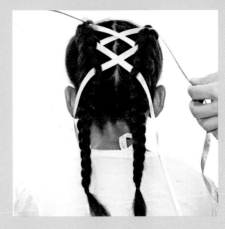

14

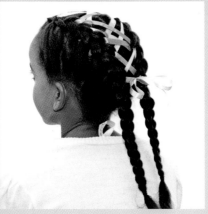

15

this process with the other side of the ribbon.

14. Repeat this entire process with another 32-inch ribbon, anchoring it at the top of the braids and then weaving it back and forth between the two braids.

15. To finish, tuck the ends of one ribbon together in a knot, and conceal the knot behind one of the braids. Tie the ends of the other ribbon in a bow. Trim the ends of both ribbons so that they are tidy.

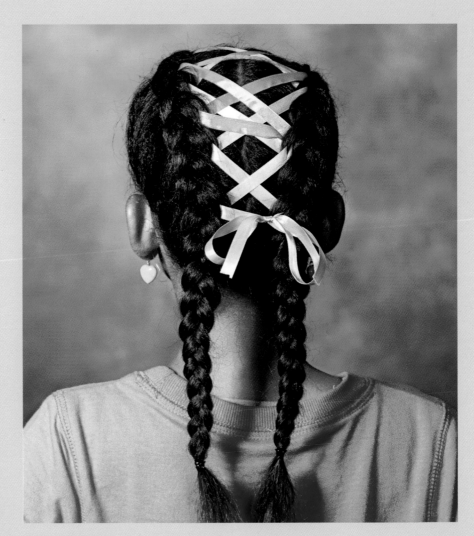

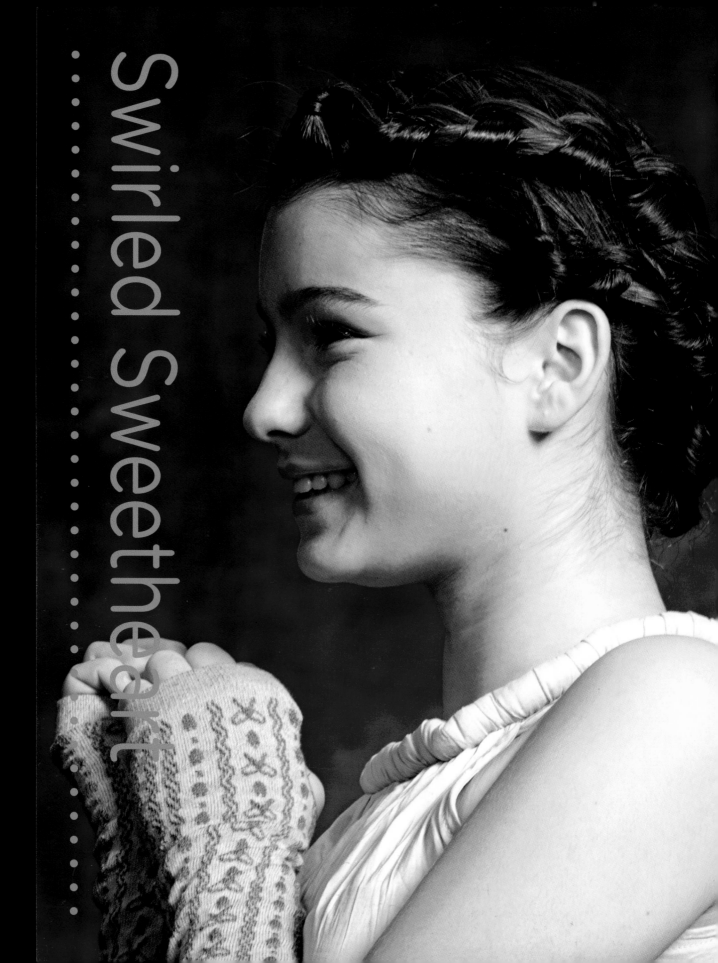

Swirled Sweetheart

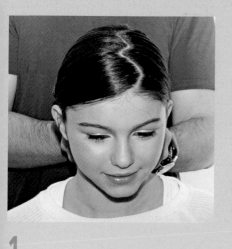

1. Wash and blow dry the hair. Rub moisturizing cream on all the hair and divide it into two sections with a zigzag part that extends from the brow to the back of the head.

2. Divide the hair on one side of the part into top and bottom sections. Hold the bottom section of hair with a clip.

3. Grasp two small sections of hair from one side of the zigzag part at the hairline.

4. Tie these sections together in a simple knot and pull the knot so that it lies close to the scalp.

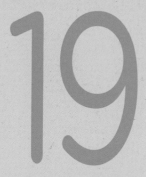

1

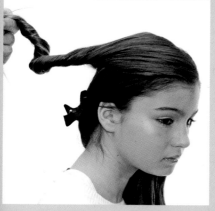

2

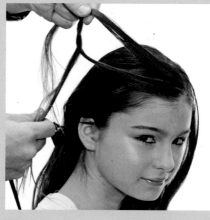

3

4

This hairstyle is sure to sweep you off your feet. It features two nicely knotted bunches of hair, swirled up and secured with a pretty pink flower.

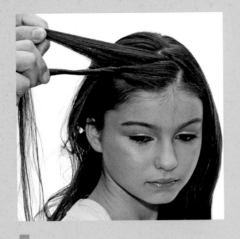

5

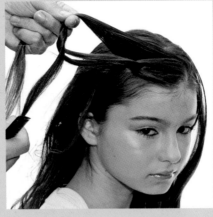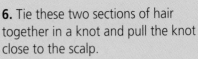

6

5. Grasp another small section of hair from this section and hold it in one hand. Hold the sections of hair you just knotted together in the other hand.

6. Tie these two sections of hair together in a knot and pull the knot close to the scalp.

7. Continue in this manner, knotting hair from the top section while working your way towards the back of the head, until you reach the other side of the head.

8. Secure the hair about 2 inches from the ends with a hair elastic.

9. Move back to the front of the head and release the hair that you secured with a hair clip in Step 2. Repeat the process of tying knots with small sections of hair as you work your way towards the back of the head.

10. Continue tying knots along the hairline in the same manner as you did with the top hair. Secure the hair about 2 inches from the ends with a hair elastic.

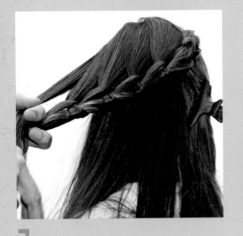

7

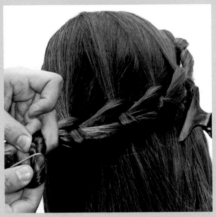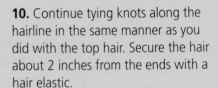

8

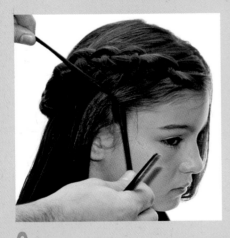

9

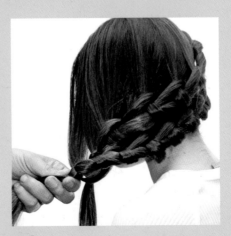

10

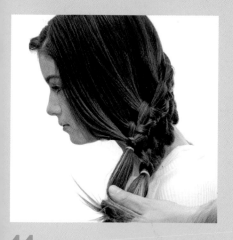

11

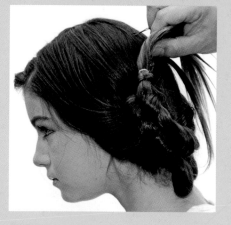

12

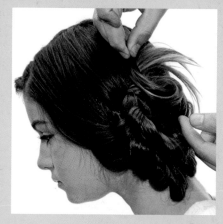

13

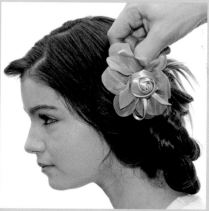

14

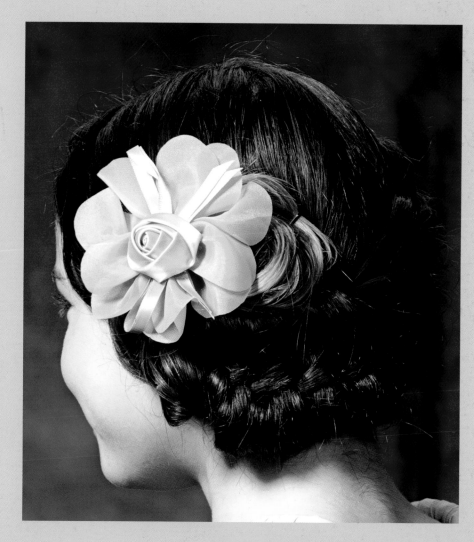

11. The two knotted bunches of hair should be parallel when they are finished.

12. Hold the bunches of hair in one hand and twist them upwards in a U shape.

13. Secure the hair at the back of the head with hair pins. Tuck the loose ends of hair into the U shape and secure with hair pins.

14. Mist with holding spray and add a flowery hair accessory.

Little Bo Sweet

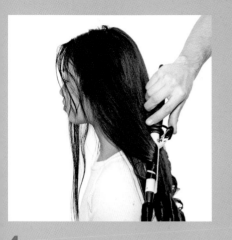

1. Wash and blow dry the hair. Curl the ends of the hair with a curling iron to make the hair a bit wavy.

2. Divide the hair into front and back sections with a part that runs from ear to ear over the crown of the head.

3. Make a middle part in the front section of hair. Weave the hair on one side of the part into a French braid.

4. Continue braiding the hair until you are about 3 inches from the ends and then secure with a hair elastic.

1

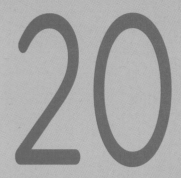

20

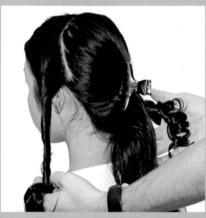

2

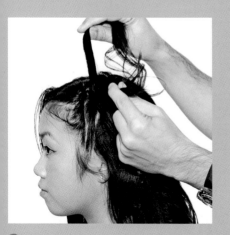

3

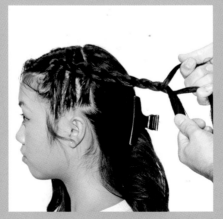

4

There's no denying it: This hairstyle is downright cute. Practice making the loops of hair a few times in advance. To get it right, you need to know the stretchiness of your hair elastics!

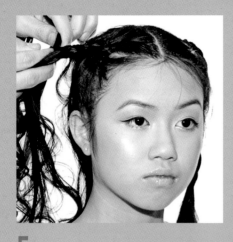

5

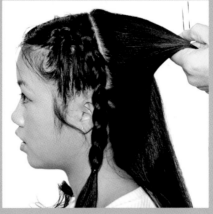

6

5. Repeat this process on the other side of the head.

6. Grasp a 2½-inch section of hair at the crown of the head just below the part.

7. Gather the hair in a ponytail and wrap a hair elastic loosely (probably twice) around the ponytail close to the scalp. Twist the hair elastic a third time and bring it around the ponytail, but this time only draw the hair partially through the elastic to create a loop of hair.

8. Pull the hair elastic a bit, twist it again, and then draw the hair through again to create another loop of hair. The final effect should resemble a bow.

9. Grasp another section of hair that's the same size as the first, and repeat the technique of creating a double loop in the hair.

10. Repeat this process to create three bow-like loops at the top back of the head.

11. Repeat it again to create two bow-like loops at the bottom of the back section, for a total of five loops.

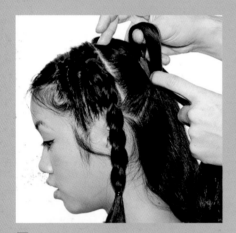

7

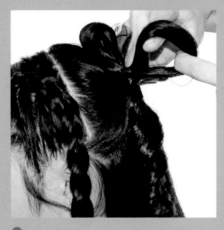

8

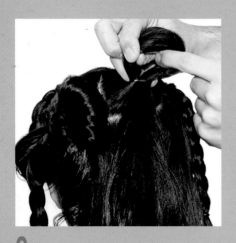

9

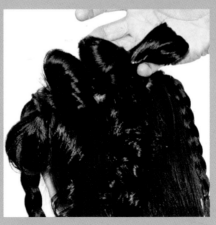

10

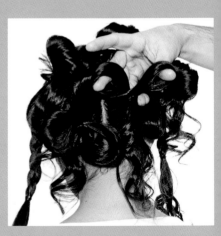

11

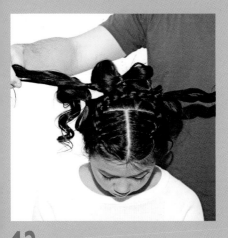

12

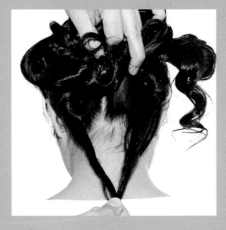

13

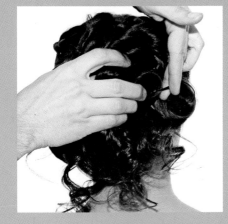

14

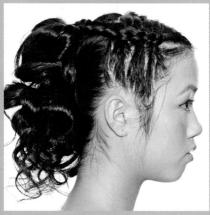

15

12. Grasp the braids and cross them in an X over the top of the head.

13. Draw the braids downwards, around the loops of hair, and connect them below the loops of hair with a hair elastic.

14. Pin the loose ends to the head with bobby pins.

15. Mist with holding spray. If you like, add a couple of bow-shaped hair accessories.

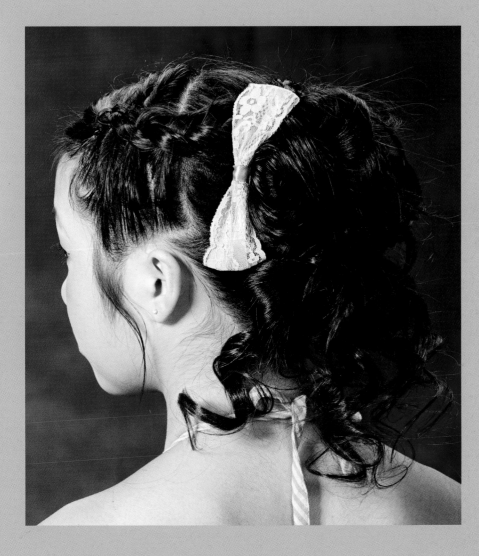

Curiously Curly

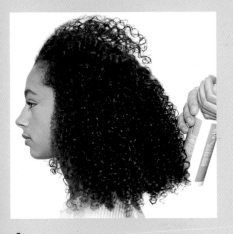

1

1. Wash the hair and rub generously with styling cream for curls. Blow dry the hair with a diffuser.

2. Gather the hair in a tight, very high ponytail.

3. Twist the hair in the ponytail and secure with bobby pins.

4. Mist the hair with hairspray. Brush the hair that's flat on the scalp to make it smooth, and blow dry.

21

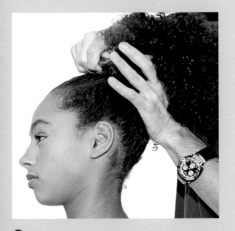

2

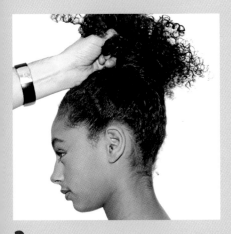

3

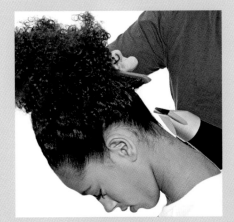

4

You'll need a hair extension for this style, so if you've never used one before, practice before the big event. You'll also need a hair ribbon that coordinates with your outfit.

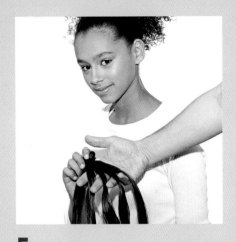

5

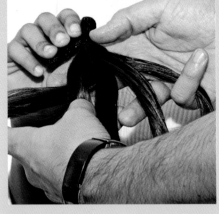

6

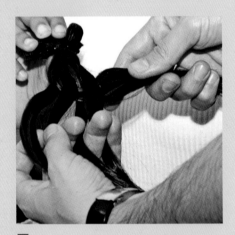

7

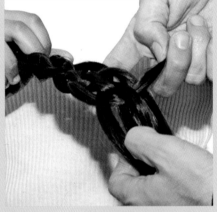

8

5. Divide the hair in the hair extension into five even sections.

6. Grasp the section on the right side of the hair extension and weave it towards the left side of the extension by bringing it under and over each adjacent section.

7. Hold the section of hair that you've just woven from the right to the left in one hand. Grasp the adjacent section of hair (the section that was previously the leftmost section of the hair extension) and bring it to the right side of the extension by weaving it under and over each adjacent section.

8. Continue in this manner until you've woven the entire hair extension.

9. Connect the hair extension to the scalp, just to the right of the ponytail base, with bobby pins.

10. Draw the hair extension over the head like a hair band and pin it on the other side of the ponytail.

11. Use a small curling iron to curl the hair in the ponytail. Curl just a small section every time, and hold each section in the curling iron for a few moments.

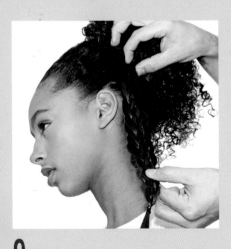

9

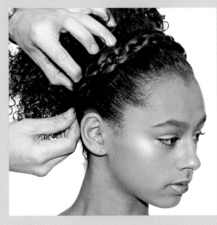

10

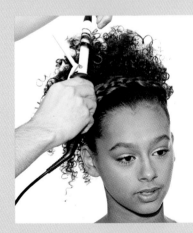

11

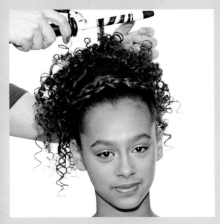

12

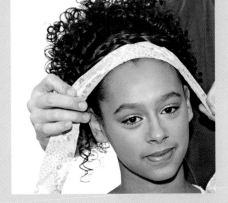

13

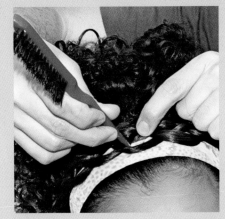

14

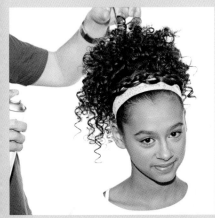

15

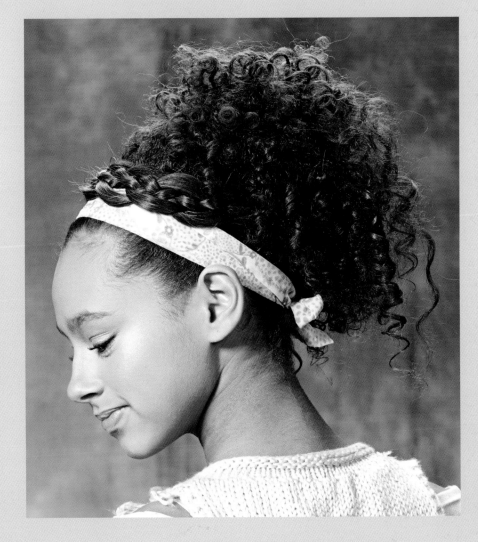

12. Repeat this to curl all of the hair in the ponytail into small, tidy curls.

13. Place a 32-inch hair ribbon along the front of the hair so that it sits right on the hairline. Let the hair ribbon hang evenly on either side and then tie the ends firmly at the back.

14. Use the end of a tail comb to draw out the hair in the hair extension a little bit, so that the top of the hair band is covered with little loops of hair.

15. Mist with holding spray.

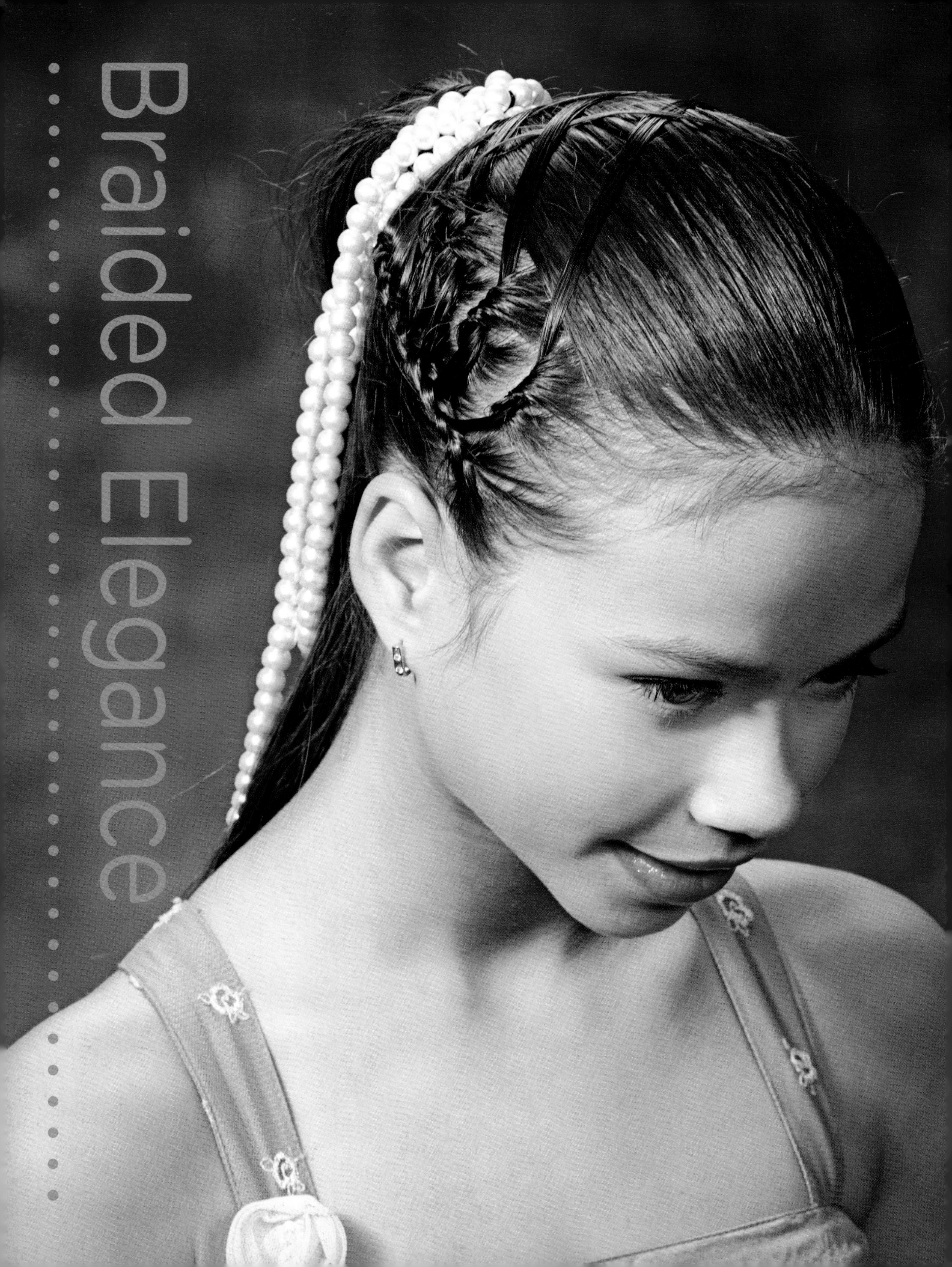
Braided Elegance

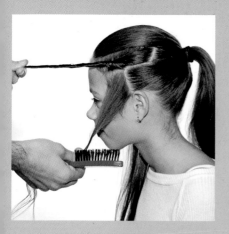

1

1. Wash and blow dry the hair. Divide the hair into three sections; one section above and in front of the left ear, one section above and in front of the right ear, and one section at the back. Rub moisturizing cream on all three sections to make them smooth. Gather the hair at the back of the head in a ponytail.

2. Secure the hair in front of the left ear in a hair clip. Grasp a 1-inch section of hair above the ear and divide it into two even sections.

3. Tie these sections together in a simple knot and let the ends of the hair hang loose.

4. Repeat this process another three times to make four simple knots in the hair above the left ear.

5. Bring the top sections of hair from each knot over the crown of the head and secure them temporarily on the other side of the head with a clip. (See photo page 94)

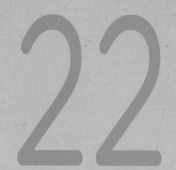

22

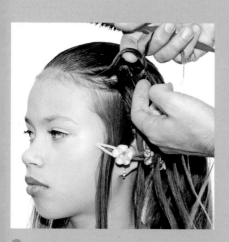

2

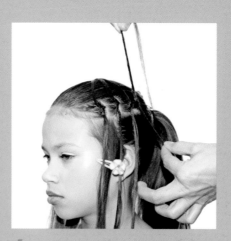

3

4

Create a decorative masterpiece by weaving braids from one side of the head to the other. It's like transforming your hair into a piece of jewelry!

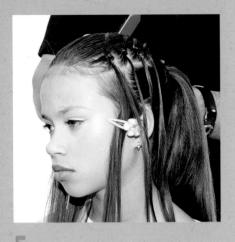

5

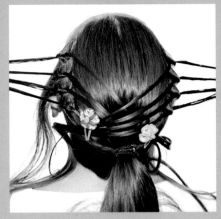

6

6. Repeat Steps 2 to 4 on the other side of the head so that you have four knots of hair on either side of the head. Of the hair extending from the knots, four sections will hang down on each side and four sections will be draped over the crown of the head.

7. Release the small section of hair at the front left side of the head and divide it into three sections. Create a simple braid that works its way towards the back of the head. As the braid moves backwards, integrate the loose sections of hair from the knots on this side of the head.

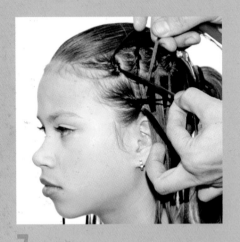

7

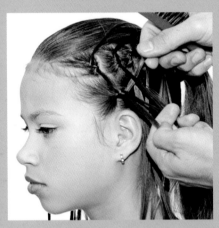

8

8. Every time you integrate a section of hair from a knot, join the section with the middle section of the braid.

9. When all four sections have been woven into the braid, secure the braid with a clip.

10. Repeat this process on the right side of the head. This time, after weaving in all the sections of hair from the knots on this side of the head, you'll start weaving in the sections of hair draped over the head from the other knots. To do this, grasp the first section of hair from the left side of the head, bring it under the 2nd and 4th sections of hair already lying across the head, and then integrate it into the braid.

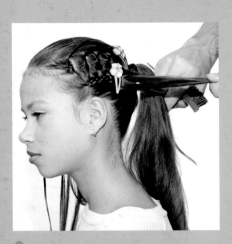

9

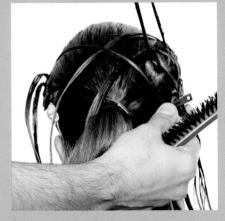

10

11. To integrate the next section of hair from the left side, bring it over the head and weave it under the 1st and 3rd sections of hair lying across the crown. Repeat Steps 10 and 11 with the next two sections of hair to create a woven look across the top of the head. Weave the braid to the end, integrating all the sections of hair from the other side.

12. Release the clip from the braid on the left side of the head and continue making the braid, integrating the hair

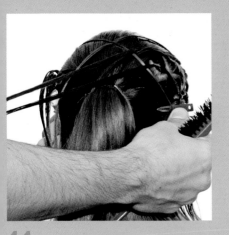

11

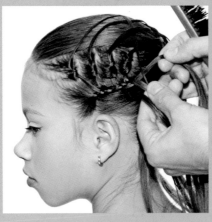

12

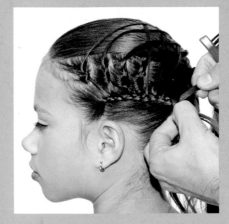

13

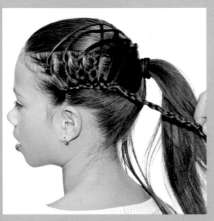

14

from the knots on the right side of the head into the braid.

13. Integrate all four sections of loose hair into the braid, one after the other.

14. Continue braiding the hair until you reach the ends and then secure the braid with a hair elastic. Roll the braid around the base of the ponytail to conceal the hair elastic and secure it with an elastic band.

15. Repeat this process on the other side of the head. Mist with holding spray.

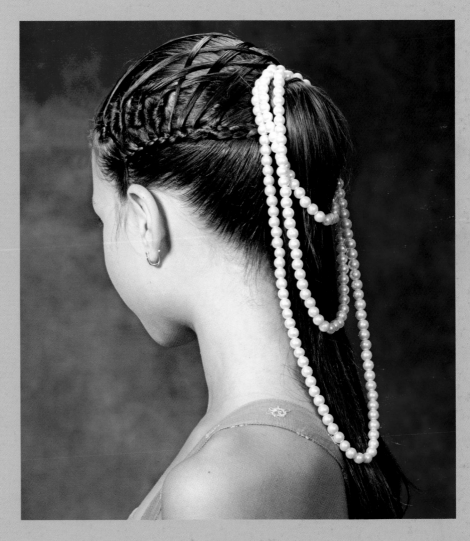

● ● ● ● ● ● ● ● ●

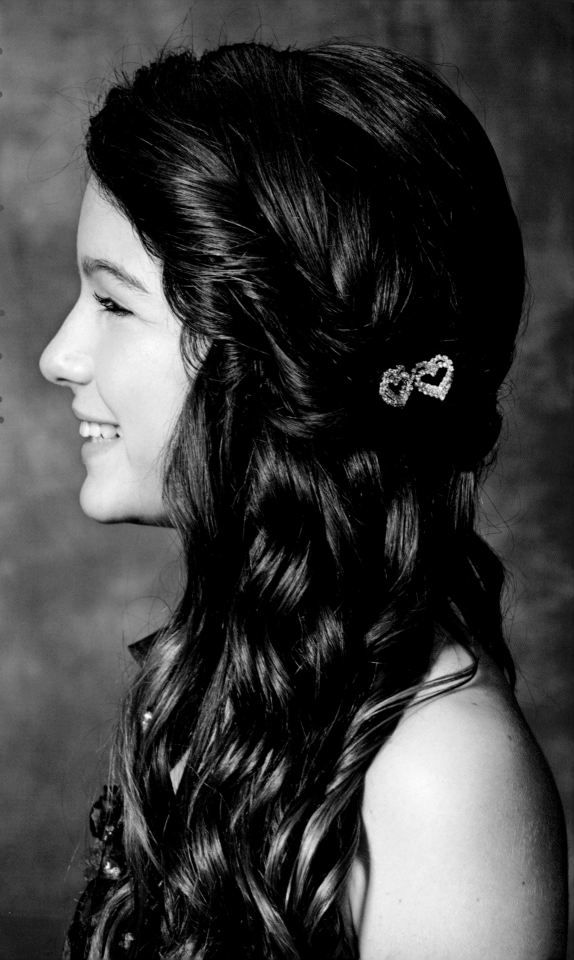

Magical Mix

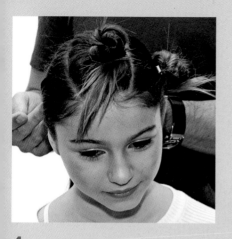

1

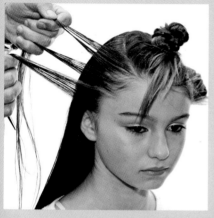

2

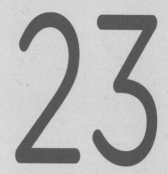

23

1. Wash and blow dry the hair. Divide the hair at the front of the head into three even sections: a middle section that extends over the crown of the head, and a section over each ear. Secure the hair in each section with a hair clip.

2. Grasp three small sections of hair from the hairline.

3. Draw the top section of hair under the middle section and then draw the bottom section under what is now the middle section.

4. Add a small section of hair from above the braid to the top section of the braid. Draw this section under the middle section to weave it into the braid, then draw the bottom section under the middle section to continue making the braid.

This design combines a bit of braiding with lots of lovely curls. It features a sweet braid on one side and loose curls on the other for a look that's fun and fanciful.

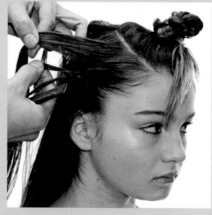

3

4

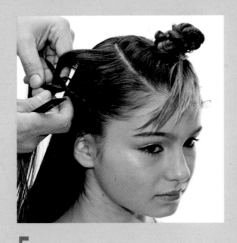

5

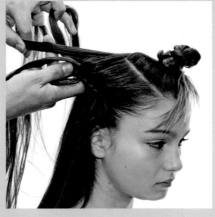

6

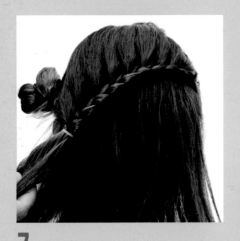

7

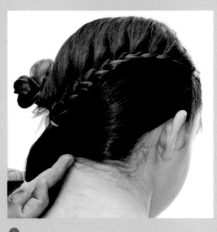

8

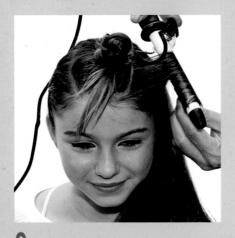
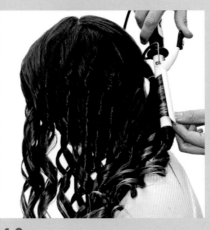

9

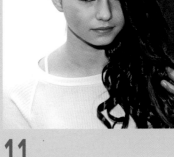

10

11

5. Continue in this manner, adding small sections of hair to the top section of the braid, as you work your way around the head.

6. Allow the braid to move in a diagonal line as it makes its way towards the right side of the head.

7. Secure the braid with a hair elastic just below the ear on the opposite side of the head.

8. Comb the hair below the braid so that it is smooth, and draw it towards the left side of the head. Secure the hair with a bobby pin under the hair elastic securing the braid.

9. Release the section of hair that you secured at the front of the left side of the head, and curl the hair with a medium curling iron.

10. Continue curling all the hair on the left side of the head.

11. Curl the section of hair at the top of the head as well.

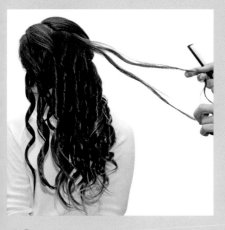

12

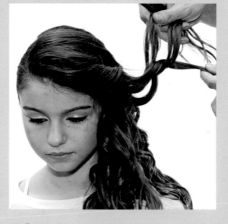

13

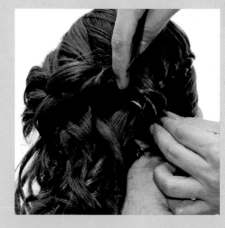

14

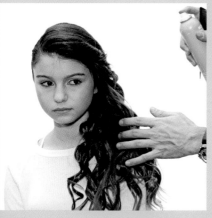

15

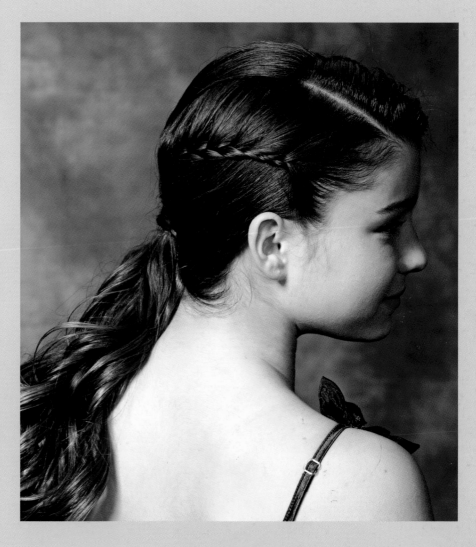

12. Run your fingers through the curls to loosen them.

13. Hold three small sections of hair from the front of the head and use them to weave a loose braid on the left side of the head.

14. Draw the braid over the hair elastic securing the first braid to conceal it, and secure with a bobby pin.

15. Mist with holding spray.

Up, Up, and Away

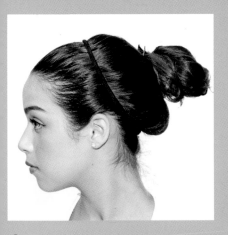

1

1. Wash and blow dry the hair. Curl all of the hair, using a curling iron, and then gather it at the back of the head in a loose ponytail. Hold the hair away from the face using an elastic hair band.

2. Place a decorative hair band over the elastic hair band and release the hair from the ponytail.

3. Make a small ponytail at the crown of the head and wrap the hair elastic close to the scalp. Loosen the hair above the hair elastic a little bit to add volume.

4. Divide the loose hair at the back of the head into four sections and secure each section with a hair elastic. Loosen the hair above the hair elastics so that there is loose hair surrounding the face. Adjust the hair elastics so that they are all evenly spaced.

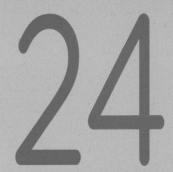

24

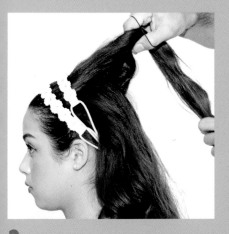

2

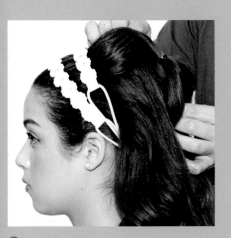

3

4

There is nothing shy about this fun hairstyle. Brimming with curls, it's just right for a fun night of frolicking with friends.

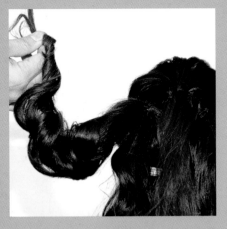

5

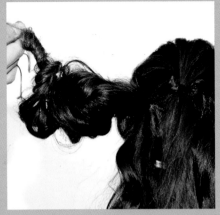

6

5. Twist one section of hair. Grasp some of the ends of the hair with one hand and push the rest of the hair upwards with the other hand to increase volume.

6. Twist the hair towards the scalp so that the volume of the hair seems to shrink.

7. Pin the hair to the scalp with hair pins. Make sure you use enough pins to secure the hair.

8. Repeat this process with the next section of hair.

9. As before, twist the hair in the ponytail, push some of it upwards with one hand, and then pin it to the scalp to create a fun, playful look.

10. Repeat this process with each section of hair, twisting the hair in a similar manner so that the hair looks deliberate, yet messy.

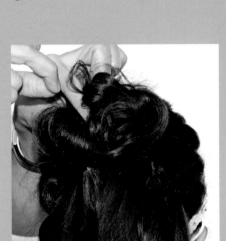

7

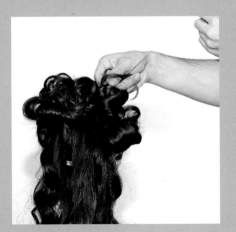

8

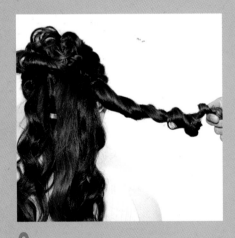

9

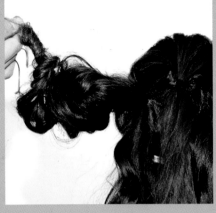

10

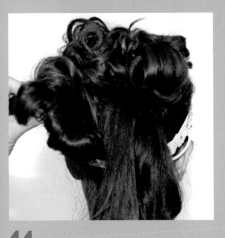

11

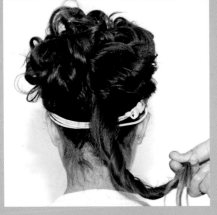

12

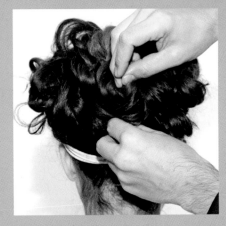

13

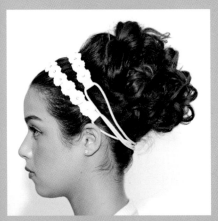

14

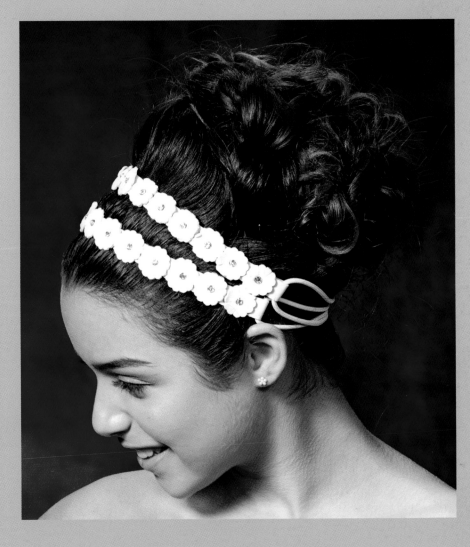

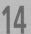**11.** To get the style just right, make sure you insert enough hair pins to hold the twists, and mist each twisted section with holding spray to secure it.

12. With just five hair elastics, a few hair pins and some finishing spray, it's possible to create a hair style that's just right for an evening out.

13. For a perfect finish, add a few more hair pins to secure the twists at the back of the head.

14. Mist with holding spray.

Zigzag Pizzazz

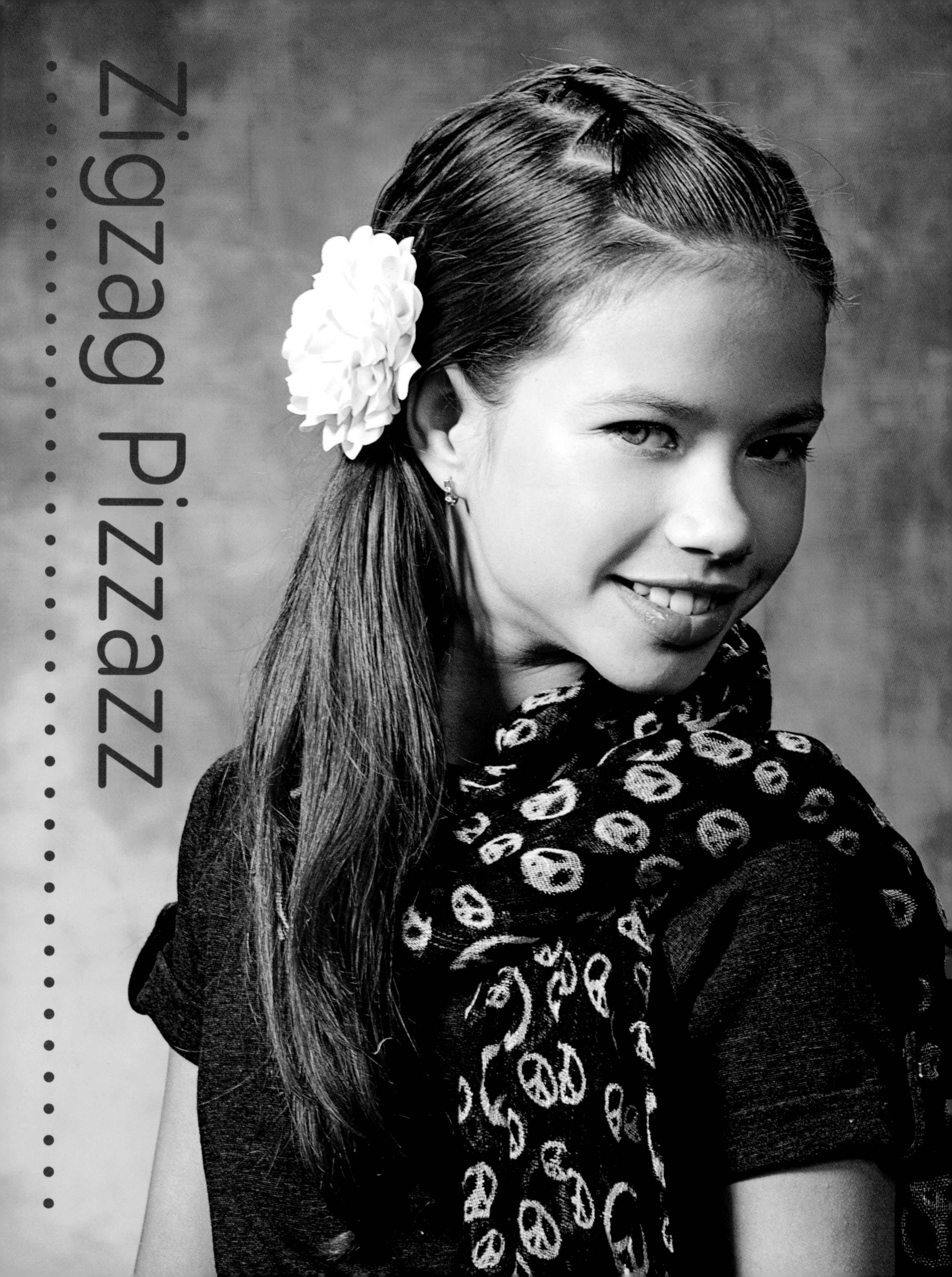

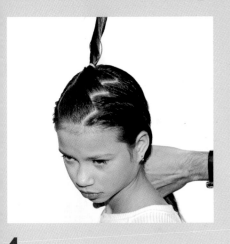

1. Wash and blow dry the hair. Make a zigzag part from the forehead to the crown of the head. Gather the hair at the top of the head in a ponytail at the crown of the head.

2. Grasp the hair at the hairline on one side of the face and divide it into top and bottom sections.

3. Grasp a section of hair on the same side of the head, adjacent to the part and the face. Twist this section of hair, draw it over the top section of hair from Step 2, and then join it with the hair in the bottom section.

4. Take a section of hair from the bottom of the head. Draw it over the bottom section of hair in Step 3 to make an X, and then join it with the hair in the top section.

5. Repeat this process, alternately taking sections of hair from the top and bottom of the head, and weaving each section into one of two main sections. (See photo page 106)

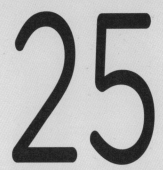

1

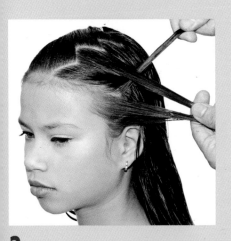

2

3

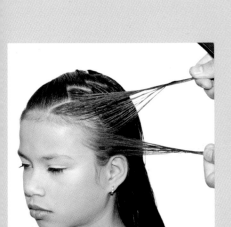

4

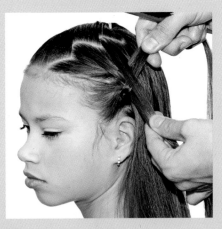

Why wait for a special occasion to create a fun hairstyle? This design is simple enough to wear to an evening at the movies with good friends. Spunky and full of pizzazz!

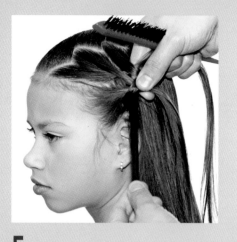

5

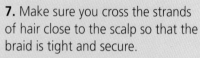
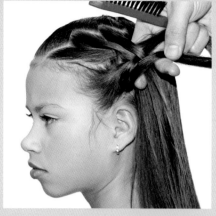

6

6. Move your way along this side of the head to make a 2-strand French braid. Rub moisturizing cream on each section of hair to create smooth, clean sections.

7. Make sure you cross the strands of hair close to the scalp so that the braid is tight and secure.

8. The sections of hair should be clearly defined so that you can see that the braid is made from sections that are woven together and increasing in size every time.

9. Continue in this manner, working your way around the back of the head and continuing on the other side. You'll also work in the ends of the hair that were collected in the ponytail.

10. Rub moisturizing cream on each section to make it more clearly defined.

11. Brush each section of hair as you add it to the 2-section braid to keep the look clean and smooth. Also make sure you keep the braid close to the scalp.

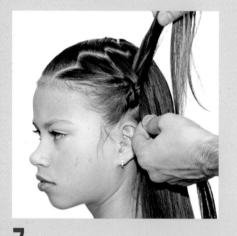

7

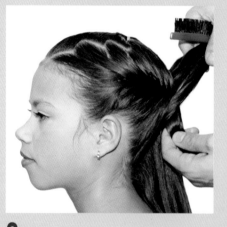

8

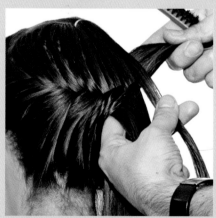

9

10

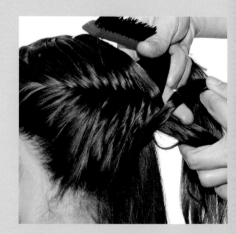

11

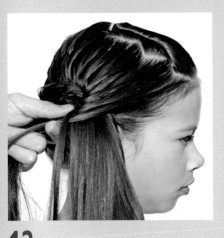

12

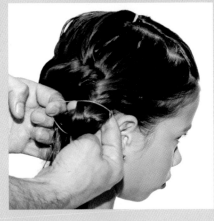

13

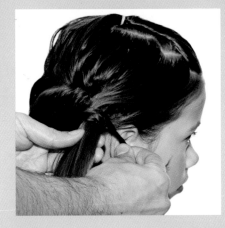

14

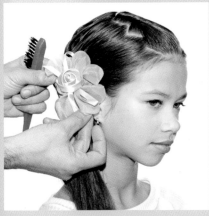

15

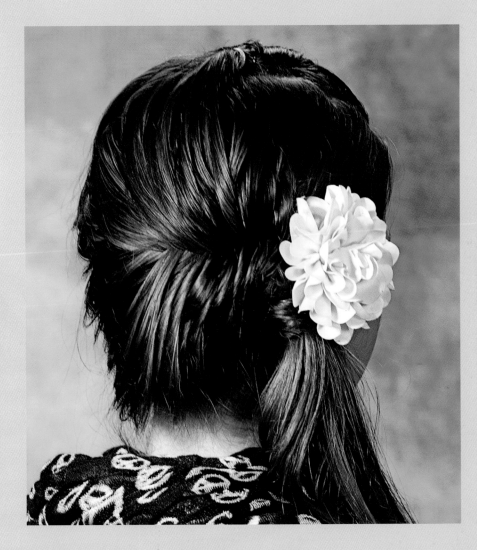

12. Continue making the braid until you've integrated all of the loose hair and have reached the ear on the other side of the head.

13. Wrap a hair elastic around the hair at the ear line to secure the braid. Leave the ends loose, as in a ponytail.

14. Wrap a section of hair in the ponytail around the hair elastic to conceal it.

15. Mist with holding spray. If you like, add a floral hair accessory for a decorative finish.

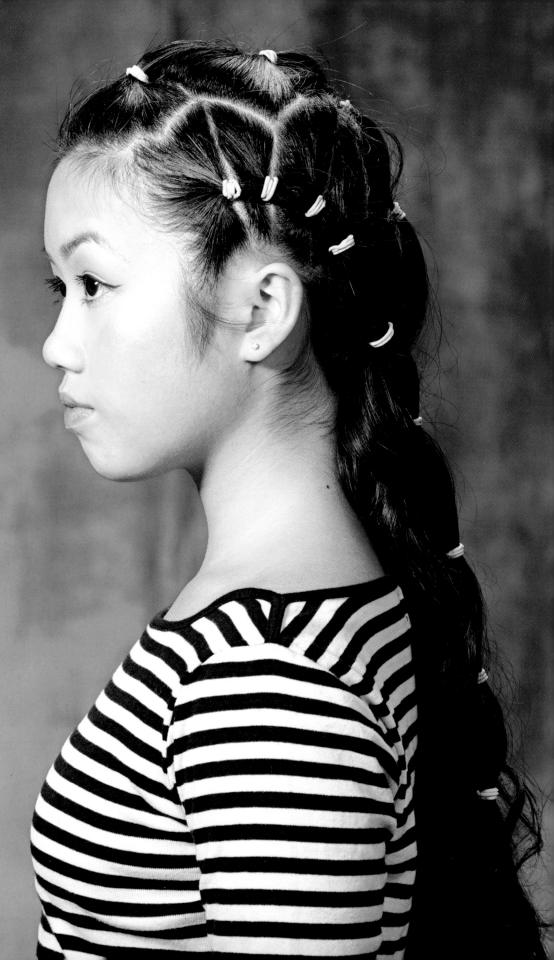

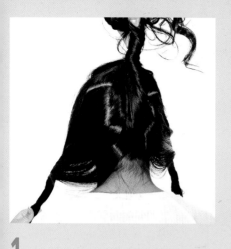

1

1. Wash and blow dry the hair. Rub moisturizing cream on all the hair and divide it into three sections: one section on the right, one on the left, and one in the middle.

2. Each section of hair should extend from the front of the head to the nape of the neck.

3. Starting with the leftmost section, grasp a ¾-inch section of hair at the hairline and secure it with a hair elastic close to the scalp.

4. Grasp another ¾-inch section of hair, immediately behind the first section.

5. Hold the two sections of hair together and secure with a hair elastic close to the scalp. (See photo page110)

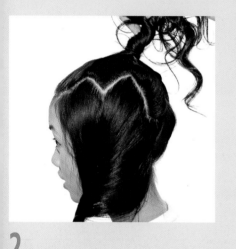

2

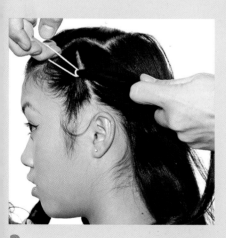

3

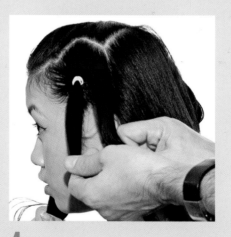

4

This simple yet striking hairstyle includes more than a dozen hair elastics. They really stand out, so make sure you like the ones that you choose.

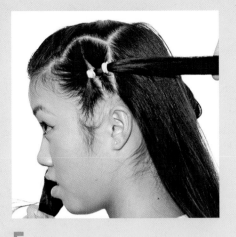

5

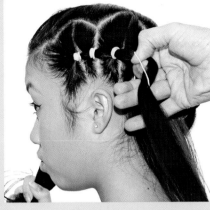

6

6. Continue in this manner, making small connected ponytails all along this side of head until you reach the nape of the neck.

7. Repeat this exact process on the other side of the head. Make sure that you place the hair elastics at the same location on both sides of the head.

8. Grasp a 1-inch section of hair from the middle section and secure it in a ponytail close to the scalp.

9. Grasp another 1-inch section of hair, immediately below the previous one, and divide it into three sections. Number these sections from 1 to 3.

10. Brush the hair in the first ponytail over the section 2 and leave the hair loose. Join sections 1 and 3 over section 2.

11. Join sections 1 and 3 in a ponytail over section 2 and the hair from the first ponytail.

12. Grasp another section of hair, immediately below the previous one, and divide it into three sections. Repeat the same process as in Step 10, connecting the side sections

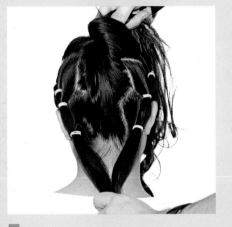

7

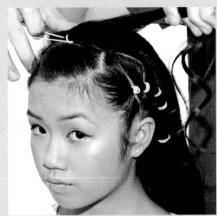

8

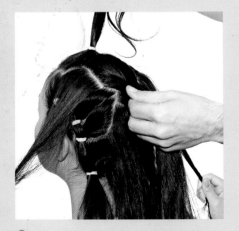

9

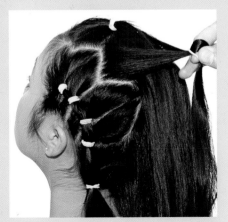

10

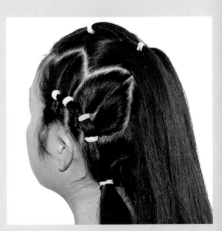

11

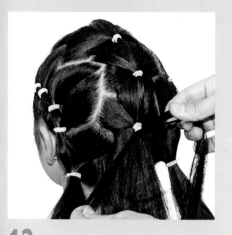

12

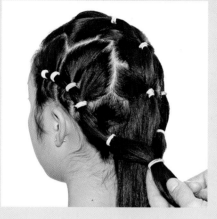

13

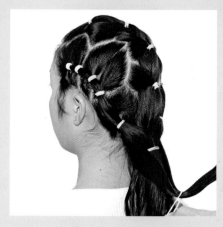

14

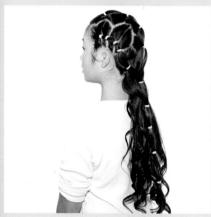

15

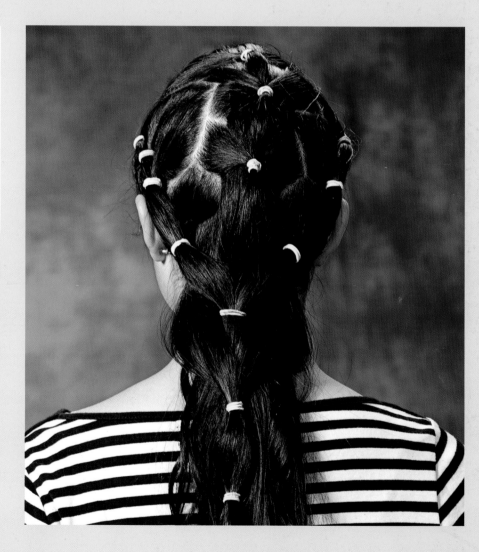

in a ponytail over the middle section, and leaving the middle section loose.

13. Repeat this process until you reach the nape of the neck, then join the ponytails at either side of the head, over the middle section of the hair, with a hair elastic.

14. Draw together a section of loose hair from each side of the head and connect them over the ponytail running down the middle.

15. To finish the hairstyle, wrap hair elastics around the ponytail running down the middle at even intervals.

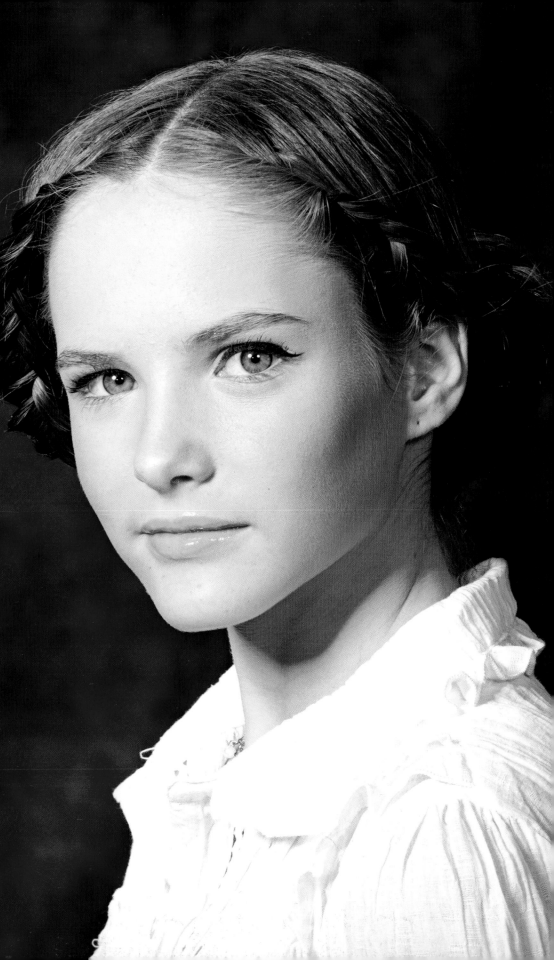

Princess Braids

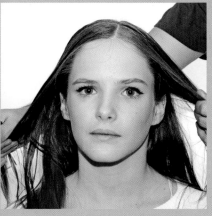

1. Wash and blow dry the hair. Make a middle part from the brow to the nape of the neck to divide the hair into two even sections.

2. Grasp a section of hair at the hairline above the left ear. Divide it into three sections and begin making a French braid.

3. Every time you weave a section of hair into the braid, integrate a bit more hair.

4. The sections of hair that you add to the braid should be about ¾-inch wide. Allow the braid to move downwards gently as it makes it way around the head.

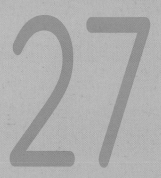

1

2

3

4

Create a curved crown of braids around the head with this simple style. It's suitable for any age or event. Just right if you've got a fantastic dress to show off!

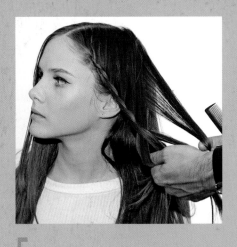

5

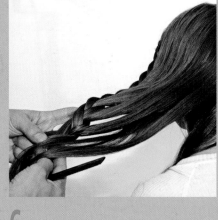

6

5. Comb out the hair sections before integrating them into the braid so that they are smooth and tidy.

6. Continue braiding the hair until you reach the part that runs down the middle of the hair. Secure the end of the braid with a hair elastic.

7. Move to the front of the hair on the other side of the head and start making another braid, using the same technique as you did for the first one.

8. Secure the end of the braid with a hair elastic.

9. Insert bobby pins in an X-shape onto each braid, a couple of inches below the crown of the head, to create a base for gathering the hair.

10. Fold up one of the braids so that the end of it is at the X of bobby pins.

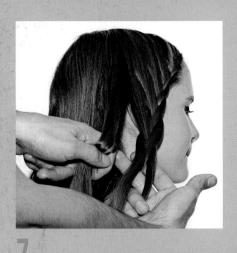

7

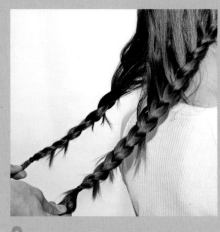

8

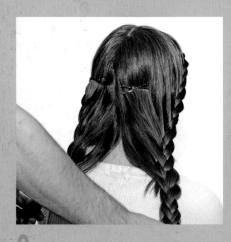

9

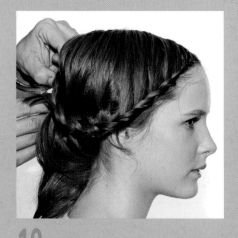

10

114

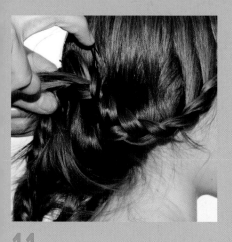

11

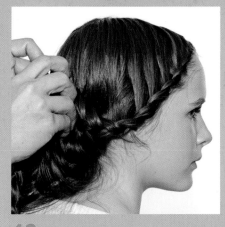

12

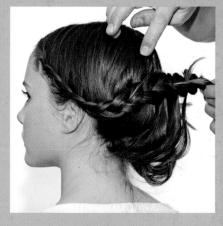

13

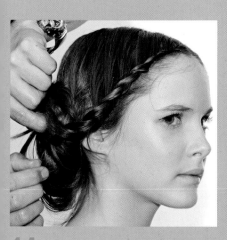

14

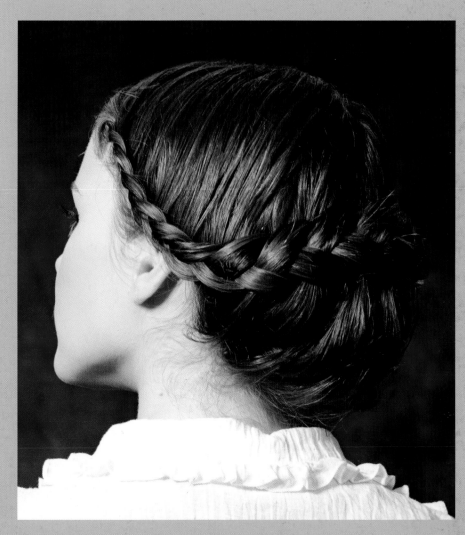

11. Secure the braid with a few bobby pins.

12. Adjust the braid so that it creates a frame for the face.

13. Repeat this process with the second braid. Tuck in the ends of the braid to conceal them and secure with hair pins.

14. Carefully draw out small sections of hair from under the braid to soften the hairstyle a bit. Mist with holding spray.

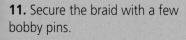

Deco by Design

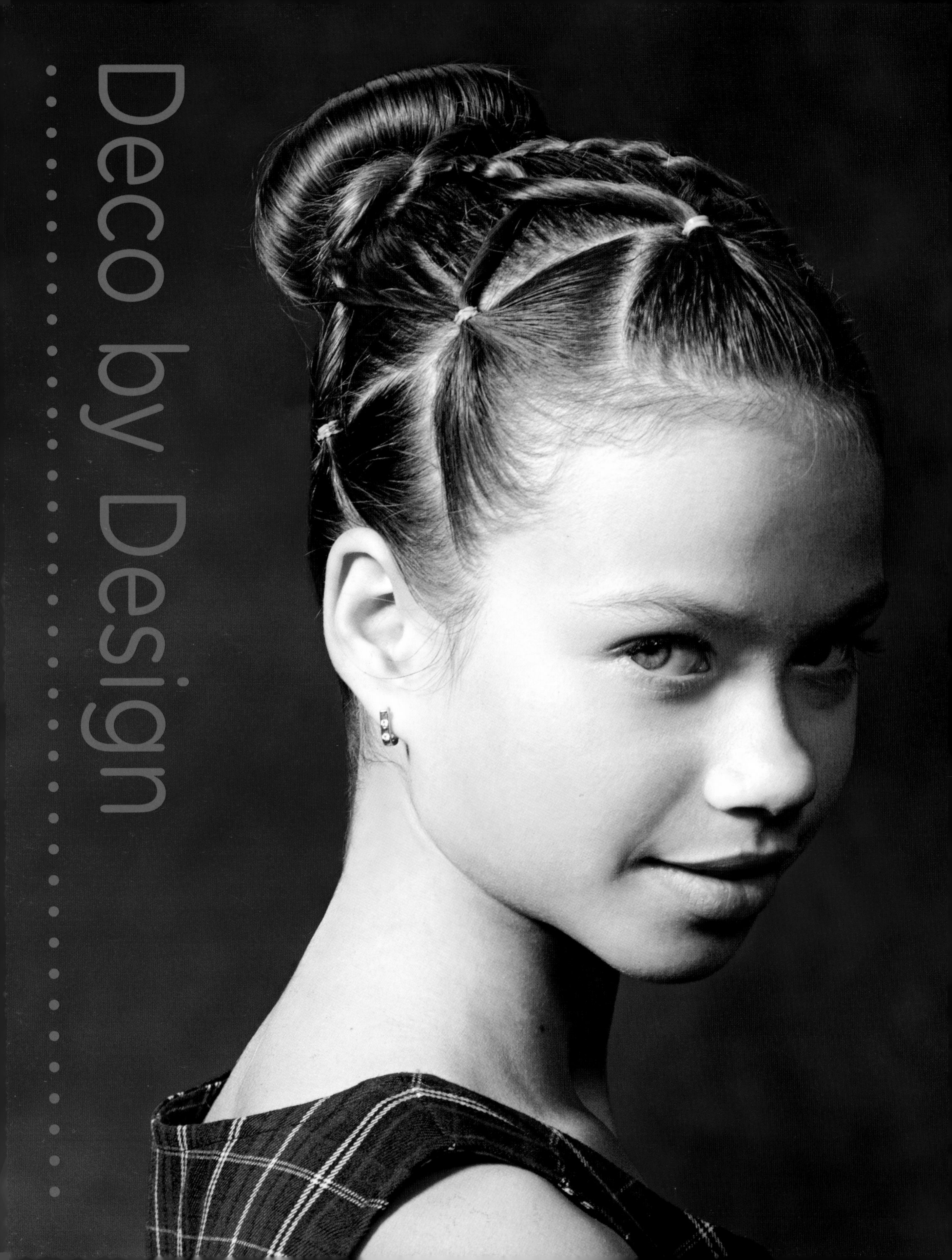

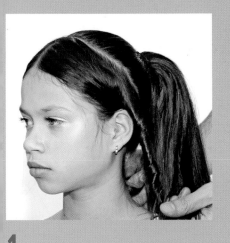

1

1. Wash and blow dry the hair. Make a part that extends from ear to ear over the crown of the head. Gather the hair behind the part in a ponytail. Make a middle part in the front section of hair.

2. Gather a triangular section of hair at the brow, with an even amount of hair coming from each side of the part. Secure this section of hair with a hair elastic.

3. Repeat this process along the hairline at the front of the head, gathering two triangular sections of hair on each side of the part. Secure each section with a hair elastic.

4. You should now have five triangular sections of hair secured with hair elastics. Number the sections from 1 to 5.

5. Divide section 3 (the middle section) into two even sections. Divide section 4 into two even sections. Draw half of section 4 over the adjacent half of section 3 to form an X. Twist the two sections together to form a rope. (See photo page 118)

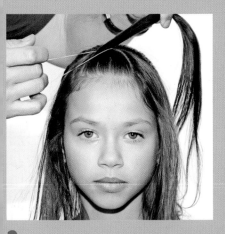

2

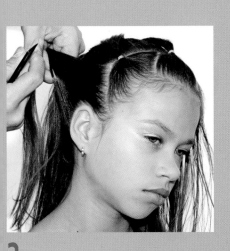

3

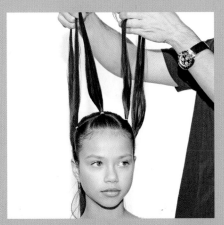

4

28

With geometric shapes at the front and a smooth, rounded back, this style is a definite head-turner. For maximum volume, you'll need a donut-shaped hair sponge.

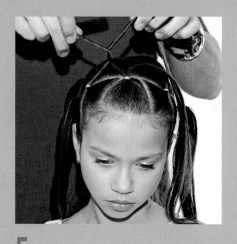

5

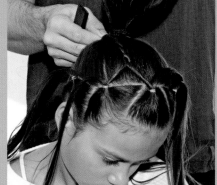
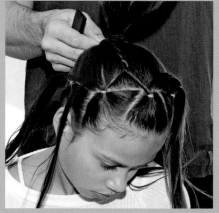

6

6. Twist these sections together into a rope until you reach the ends of the hair. Wrap the twisted rope of hair around the base of the ponytail you made in Step 1.

7. Divide section 2 into two even sections and draw the section that's adjacent to section 3 over the loose half of section 3 to form an X. Twist the sections together into a rope until you reach the ends of the hair, and then wrap the twisted rope around the base of the ponytail. Repeat this process by twisting together all of section 1 with half of section 2, and all of section 5 with half of section 4.

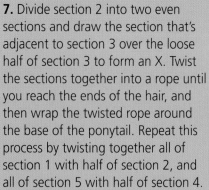

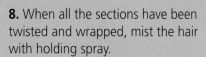

8. When all the sections have been twisted and wrapped, mist the hair with holding spray.

9. Take the donut-shaped hair sponge that matches the color of the hair.

10. Draw the ponytail through the middle of the sponge and draw the sponge down until it reaches the head.

11. Brush the hair in the ponytail in every direction so that it covers the entire sponge.

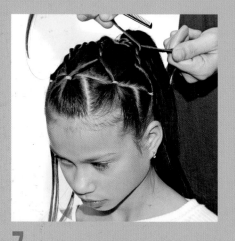

7

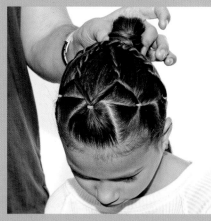

8

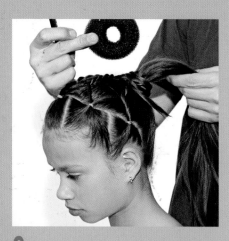

9

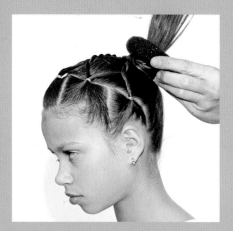

10

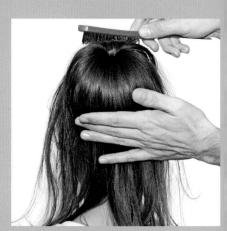

11

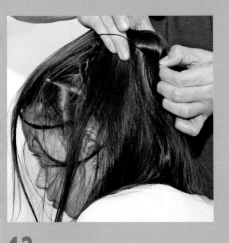

12

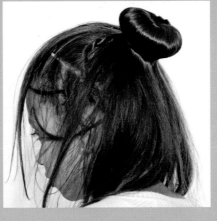

13

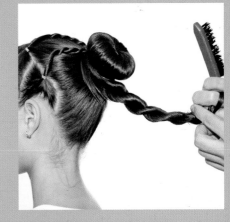

14

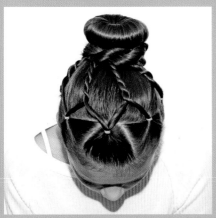

15

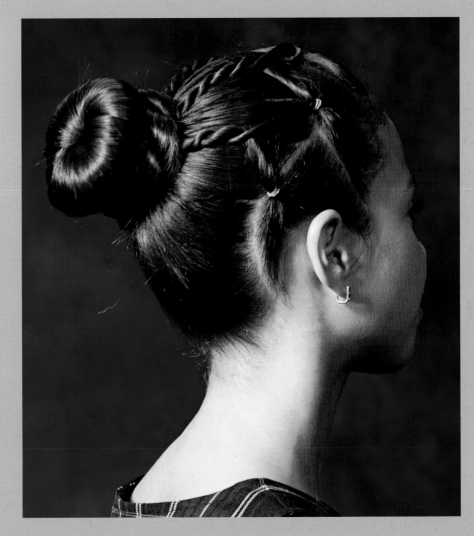

12. Wrap a hair elastic over the hair, securing it around the sponge.

13. You will now have a smooth donut-shaped ponytail.

14. Divide the hair extending from the ponytail into two even sections at the top of the ponytail. Wrap the sections around the ponytail so that they meet at the bottom and then twist the sections together to form a rope.

15. Wrap the hair rope around the base of the ponytail and secure with bobby pins. Mist with holding spray.

Soulful Sister

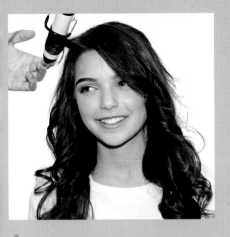

1

1. Wash the hair, style it with a bit of mousse, and then blow dry it. Curl all of the hair with a medium curling iron.

2. Gather a section of hair at the top of the crown.

3. Draw out one section of hair on each side of the section that's gathered on the top of the head, and secure with hair clips.

4. Brush the center section of hair forward and secure with a pair of bobby pins, inserting them in an X-shape. Mist with a bit of hair spray.

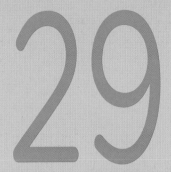

29

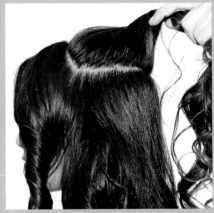

2

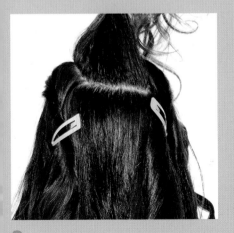

3

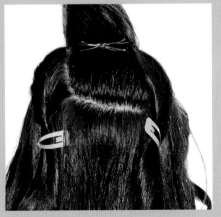

4

Get soulfully sweet with this design. You'll need a round hair extension to create the volume in this free-flowing hairstyle.

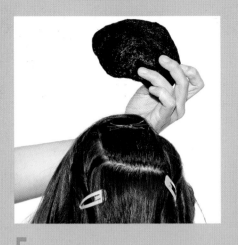

5

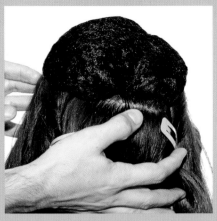

6

5. To create a lush and full-volume look, you'll need a round hair extension.

6. Secure the hair extension on the top of the head using hair pins. Make sure you insert the pins close to the scalp.

7. Gently brush back the section of hair that you brushed forward in Step 4 so that it completely covers the hair extension.

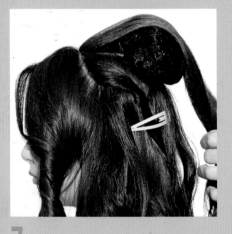

7

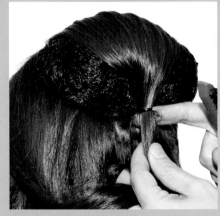

8

8. Draw out a section of hair located near the front left side of the hair extension and bring it to the back of the head. Join this section of hair and the hair that was pulled over the extension with a small hair elastic to keep the hair covering the extension in place.

9. Release one of the sections of hair that you secured in Step 3 and gently brush it over the hair extension, covering this side of the extension completely. Mist with hair spray.

10. Draw the hair to the other side of the extension. Try to create a cover for the extension that is tidy and smooth.

11. Secure the hair just below the hair extension with a hair pin.

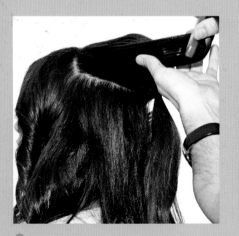

9

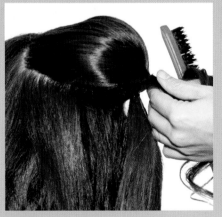

10

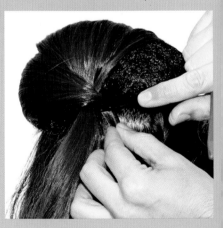

11

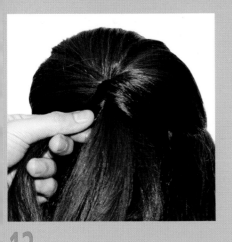

12

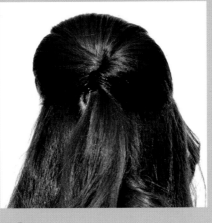

13

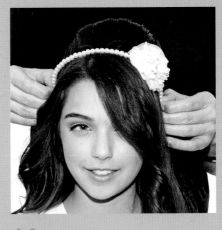

14

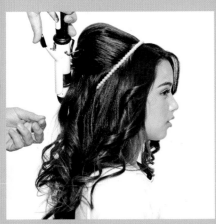

15

12. Repeat this process with the other section of hair that you set aside in Step 3. Gently brush out the hair, bring it over the hair extension, and pin it on the other side.

13. At this point, you've created a lush base at the top of the head, using a hair extension, hair elastic, and a couple of hair pins.

14. For extra elegance, add a flowery pearl hair band.

15. If any of the curls have come loose during the styling, re-curl them with the curling iron and mist with holding spray.

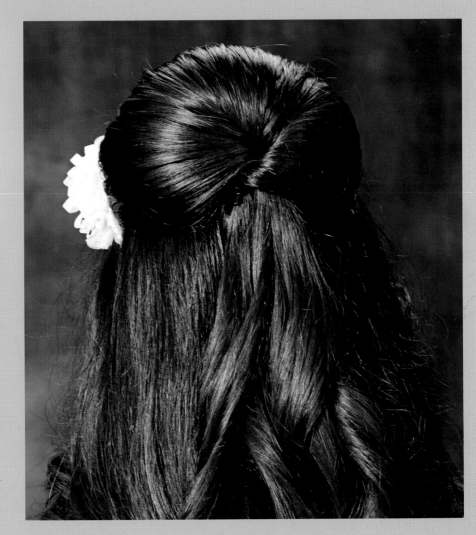

Sweep Me Sideways

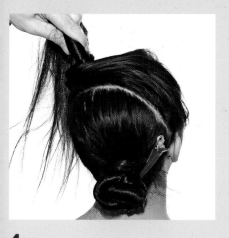

1

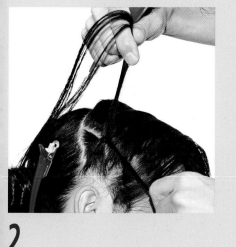

2

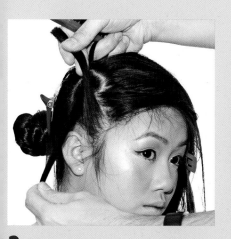

3

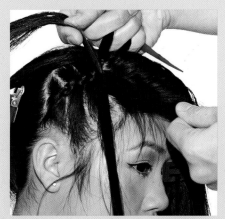

4

1. Wash and blow dry the hair. Rub moisturizing cream on all the hair and then divide it into front and back sections with a part that runs from ear to ear over the crown of the head. Secure the back section in a low ponytail.

2. Draw out a small section of hair above one ear, divide it into three sections, and begin making an inside-out French braid. This means you'll be passing the left and right sections of hair under the middle section, rather than over it.

3. Add a small section of hair to each left and right section as you make the braid.

4. Continue braiding the hair, working your way towards the front of the head. Make sure the sections are tidy and clearly defined so that the braid really stands out.

5. Continue braiding the hair, including most of the hair at the front of the face. Leave a few strands of hair loose to soften the look and frame the face. (See photo page 126)

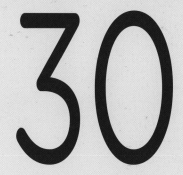

30

Add body and volume to straight hair with this pretty side braid. The braid protrudes a bit from the head in a technique known as an inside-out French braid. It's made by passing the left and right sections of hair under the middle section rather than over it.

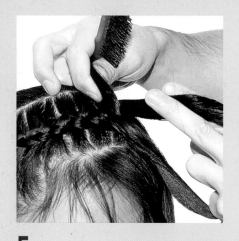

5

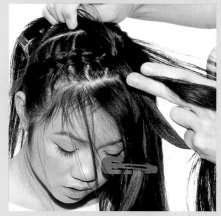

6

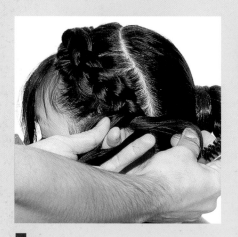

7

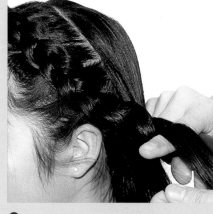

8

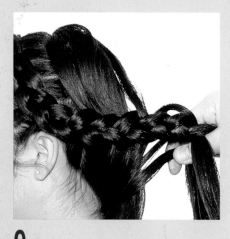

9

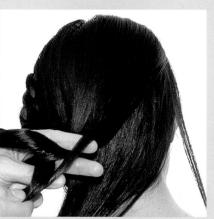

10

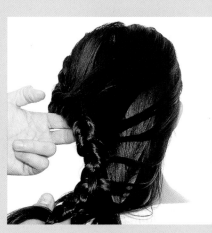

11

6. At every stage of the braid, you'll hold one section of hair in each hand and have one section in the middle, to which you'll add hair with every phase of the weave.

7. Make sure the braid stays close to the scalp. Continue braiding over the top of the head and around the face, until you reach the other ear.

8. Continue weaving the braid. When you've used all the hair that was in the top section of hair, release the ponytail at the back of the head and start integrating this hair into the braid as well.

9. The braid will still be an inside-out French braid, but will no longer be close to the scalp.

10. Continue adding small sections of hair to the braid with every weave. At this stage, the braid will be on the back left side of the head, but you'll be integrating sections of hair from the back right side.

11. You should be able to see small sections of hair that connect to the braid, one after the other.

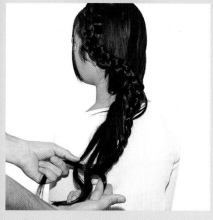

12

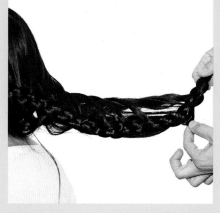

13

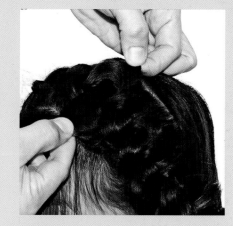

14

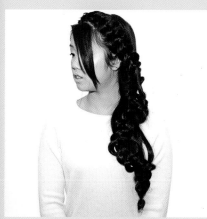

15

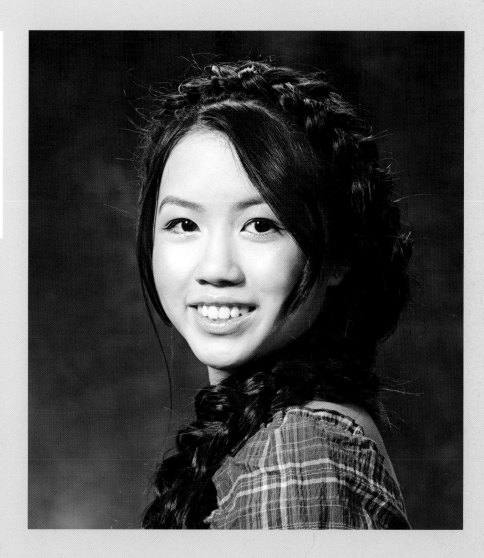

12. It's important to add sections of hair from the hairline and then from the back of the head.

13. When you reach the end of the hair, secure the braid with a hair elastic. Loosen the braid a little by gently tugging on strands of hair.

14. Be very gentle when you tug on the hair. You want to increase the volume of the braid but don't want the braid to look messy.

15. Let the braid hang down one shoulder and mist with holding spray.

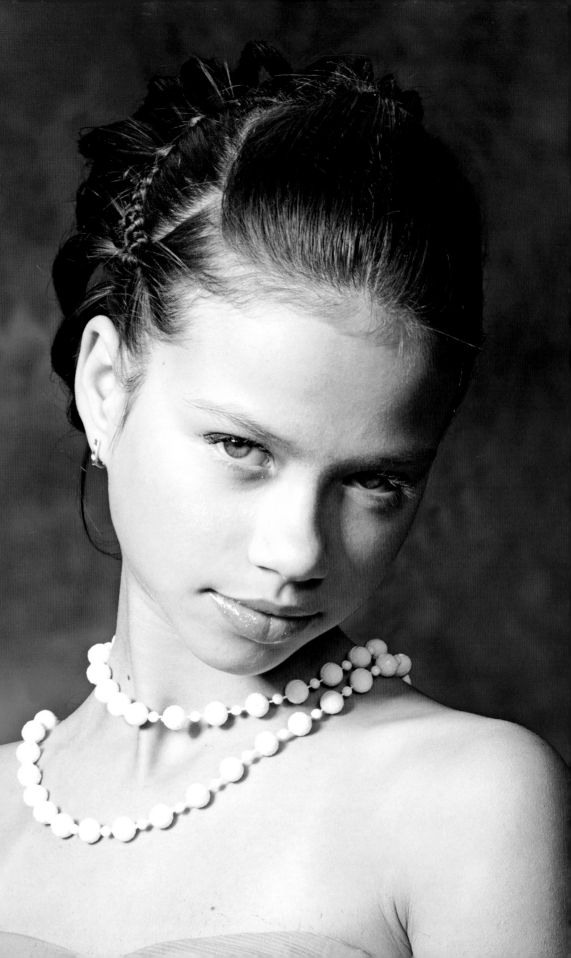

Fantastical Fountain

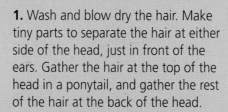

1. Wash and blow dry the hair. Make tiny parts to separate the hair at either side of the head, just in front of the ears. Gather the hair at the top of the head in a ponytail, and gather the rest of the hair at the back of the head.

2. Divide the small section of hair at the right side of the head into three even sections and start making a braid.

3. Continue braiding the hair to form a small, tight braid.

4. Grasp one of the sections of hair in the braid and push the other two sections towards the root to make the braid even tighter. Secure the end of the braid to the ponytail at the back of the head with bobby pins.

31

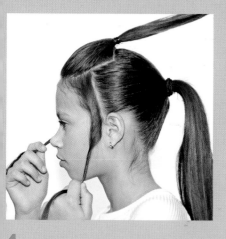

1

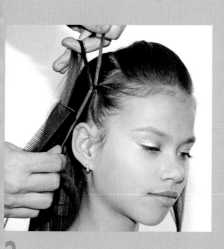

2

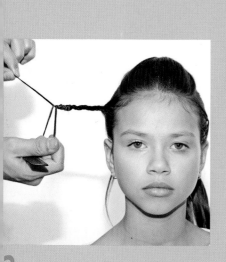

3

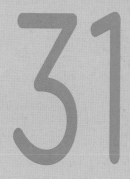

4

This artistic hairstyle looks wonderfully delicate, but is actually quite secure. This means you can wear it to any affair and really have fun with it!

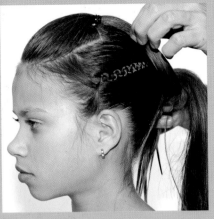

5

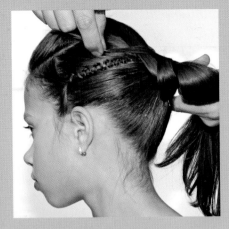

6

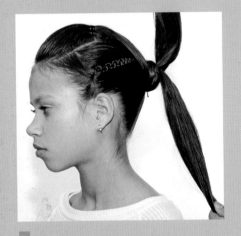

7

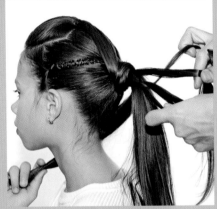

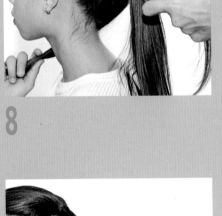

8

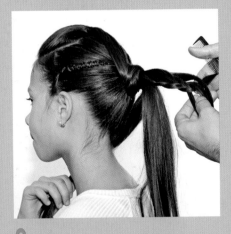

9

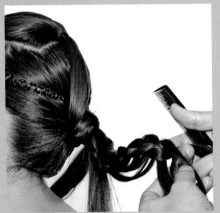

10

5. Make a similar braid on the left side of the head and secure it to the ponytail at the back of the head.

6. Draw the hair gathered at the top of the head backwards, wrap it around the base of the ponytail, and secure with bobby pins.

7. Divide the ponytail at the back of the head into two even halves.

8. Set aside the right half of the ponytail for later styling, and grasp the left half in your hand. Grasp a section of hair from the right side of the ponytail section you are holding. This section should be about one-fifth the size of this ponytail half. Divide it into 3 even sections and begin making a braid.

9. Every time you weave in the right-most section of the braid, add a small section of hair from the rest of this ponytail half.

10. Continue braiding the hair in this half of the ponytail. Since you are adding hair to one side of the braid only, the hair you add will really stick out.

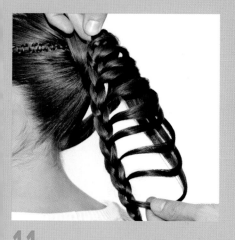

11

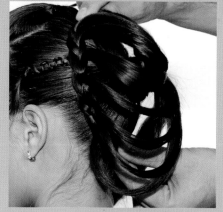

12

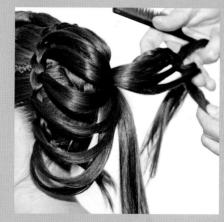

13

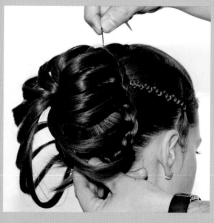

14

11. When you reach the end of the braid, secure it with a hair elastic. You should be able to clearly see the sections of hair that are connected along the braid.

12. Fold the braid forwards and secure with hair pins.

13. Repeat the same technique with the hair on the other side of the ponytail.

14. Secure the braid to the scalp with bobby pins. Mist with holding spray.

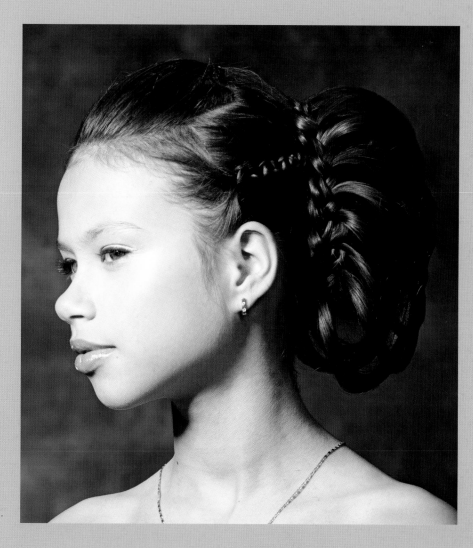

• • • • • • • • • •

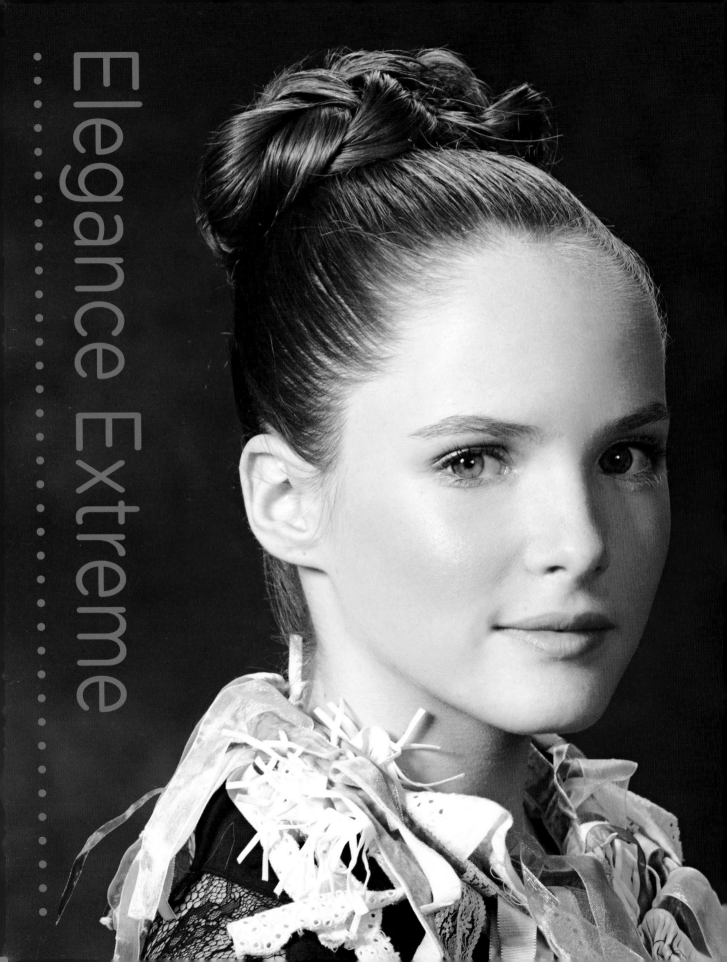

Elegance Extreme

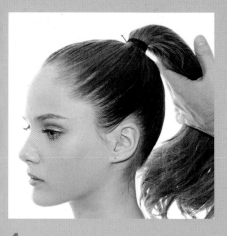

1

1. Wash and blow dry the hair. Gather all of the hair at the top of the head in a high ponytail.

2. Draw a small section of hair from the ponytail and wrap it around the hair elastic to conceal it.

3. Grasp one-quarter of the ponytail in your hand and rub it with moisturizing cream so that it is smooth and easy to style. Wrap the hair around itself to form a loop and then pull the end of the hair through the loop to make a simple knot.

4. Hold the hair close to the root while pulling the ends to tighten the knot.

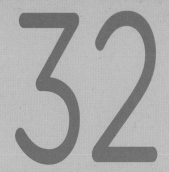

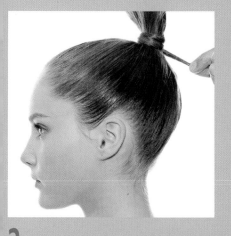

2

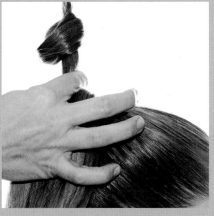

3

4

Here's a hairstyle that's full of character. Tightly pulled around the face and playfully braided at the top, it definitely demands attention.

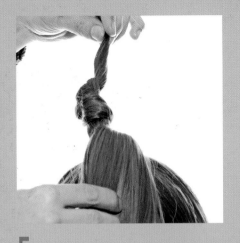

5

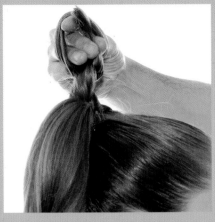

6

5. When the knot is tight, draw this section of hair forward and secure temporarily with a hair clip.

6. Grasp another section of hair that is similar in size and tie it in a simple knot. Pull the hair to secure the knot and then temporarily secure the knot to the head with a hairclip.

7. Repeat this process to make two more knots that are similar in size.

8. You should now have four sections of knotted hair that are temporarily secured to the scalp.

9. Release the clips from all four sections of hair and hold the sections together in your hand.

10. Bring the sections together at the back of the head and secure the ends with a hair elastic.

11. Hold the ends of the hair and draw the knots forward around the base of the ponytail.

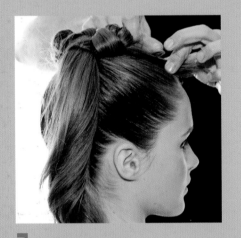

7

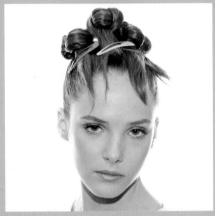

8

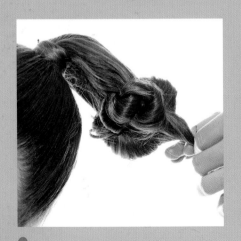

9

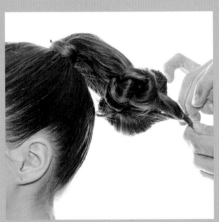

10

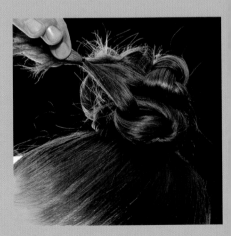

11

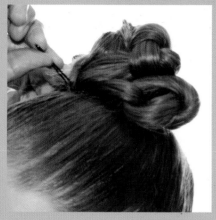

12

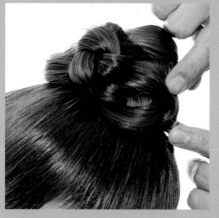

13

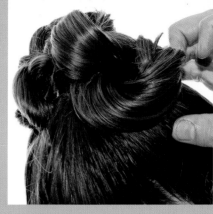

14

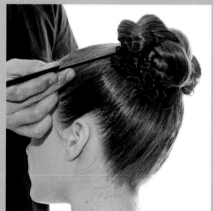

15

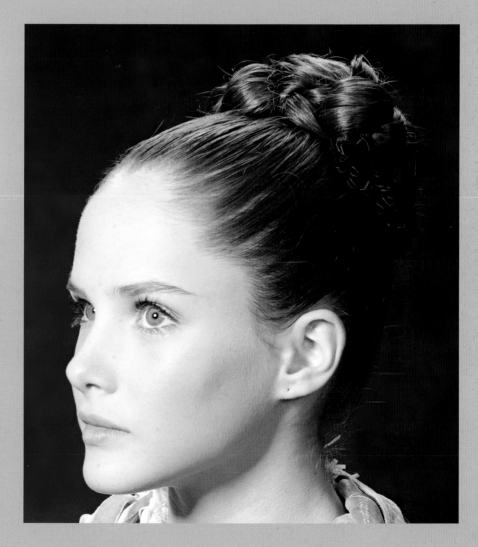

12. Secure the hair elastic at the end of the knotted sections at the base of the ponytail with bobby pins.

13. Arrange the knots all around the ponytail base and secure them with bobby pins.

14. Rubbing the hair with moisturizing cream makes it easy to shape so that the knotted hair looks just right.

15. Mist with holding spray. Add a few decorative hair clips, if you like.

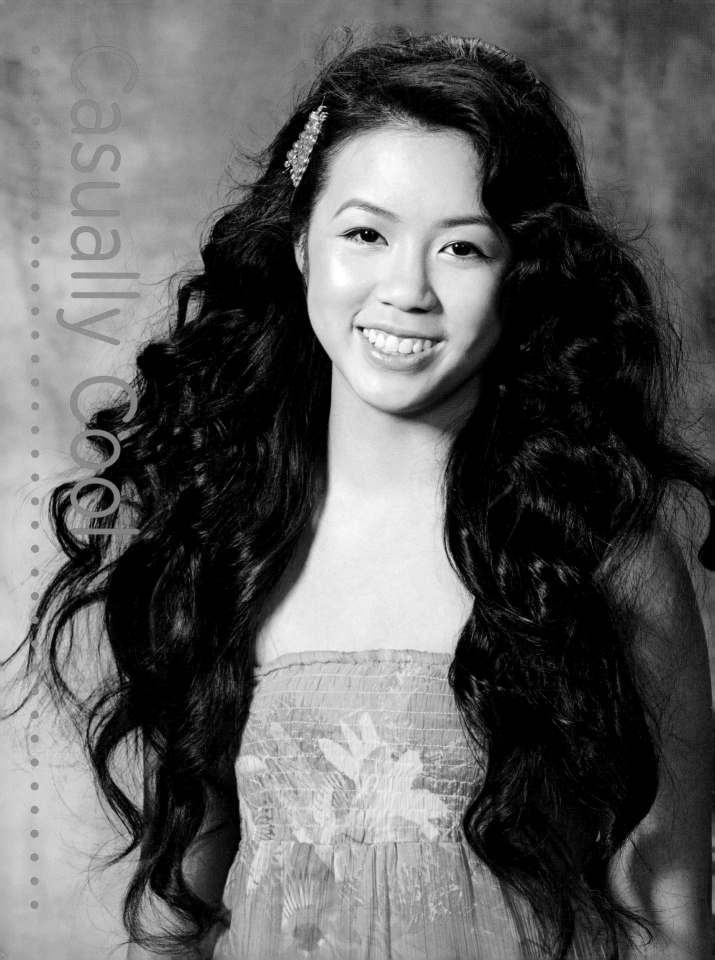

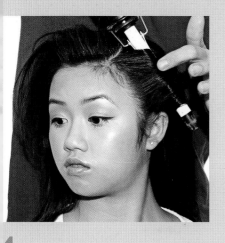

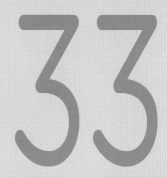
1. Wash the hair, rub it with a bit of styling mousse, and then blow dry it. Curl it with a small curling iron.

2. To create curls that hold, mist each section of hair with styling spray before rolling it with the curling iron. Hold the iron for a few seconds on each curl.

3. Because you're working with a small curling iron, use large sections of hair each time to create a look that is rich in volume.

4. Make a side part above the left eyebrow and continue curling the hair all over the head.

1

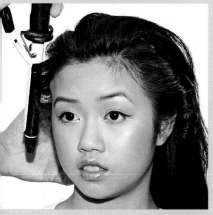

2

Just because you usually have pin-straight hair, it doesn't mean you always have to have flat hair! Adding waves is easy, fun, and a perfect way of dressing up casually cool for a special occasion.

3

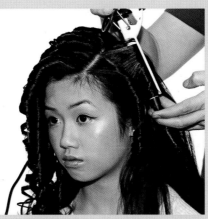

4

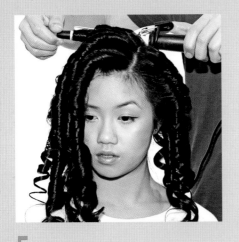

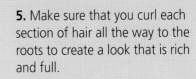

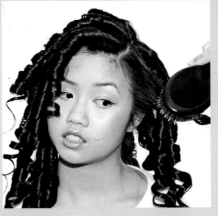

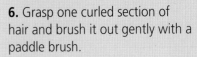

5. Make sure that you curl each section of hair all the way to the roots to create a look that is rich and full.

6. Grasp one curled section of hair and brush it out gently with a paddle brush.

7. Repeat Step 6 to brush out all of the curled sections of hair.

8. Continue brushing the hair until it is all wavy.

9. After all of the curls have been brushed into waves, mist the brush with a bit of hair spray and brush out the waves again.

10. After each section is brushed out, mist the hair brush again with a bit more styling spray and then brush a larger section of hair.

11. Mist all the hair from a distance of about 8 inches.

5

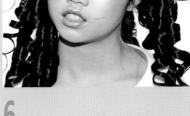

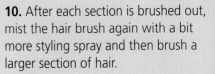

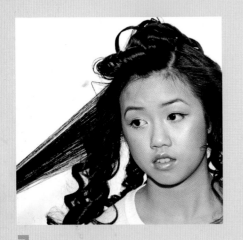

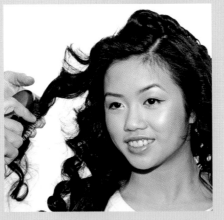

6

7

8

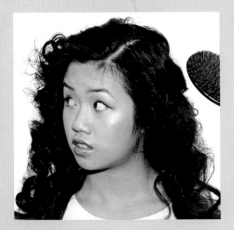

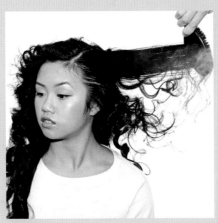

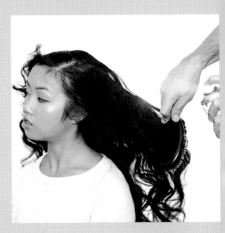

9

10

11

138

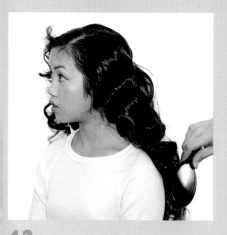

12

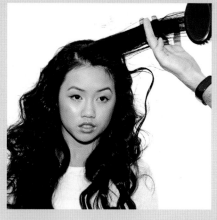

13

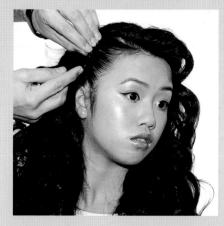

14

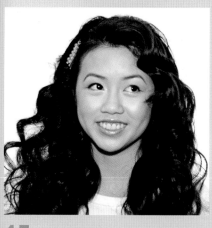

15

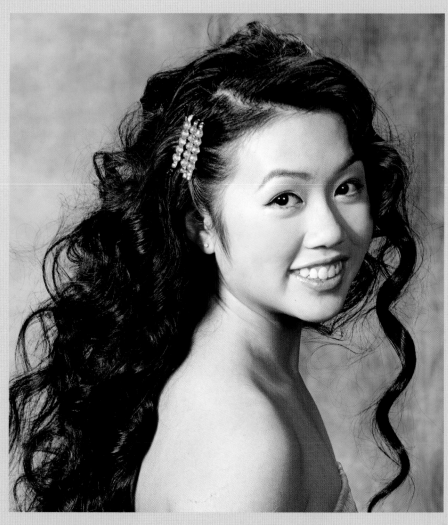

12. Every time you brush out the hair, the waves become larger and richer.

13. To create volume at the forehead, backcomb the bangs at the roots.

14. Gather the hair at one side of the head and secure with bobby pins close to the scalp.

15. Add pretty hair accessories on top of the bobby pins to hide the pins and dress up the hairstyle.

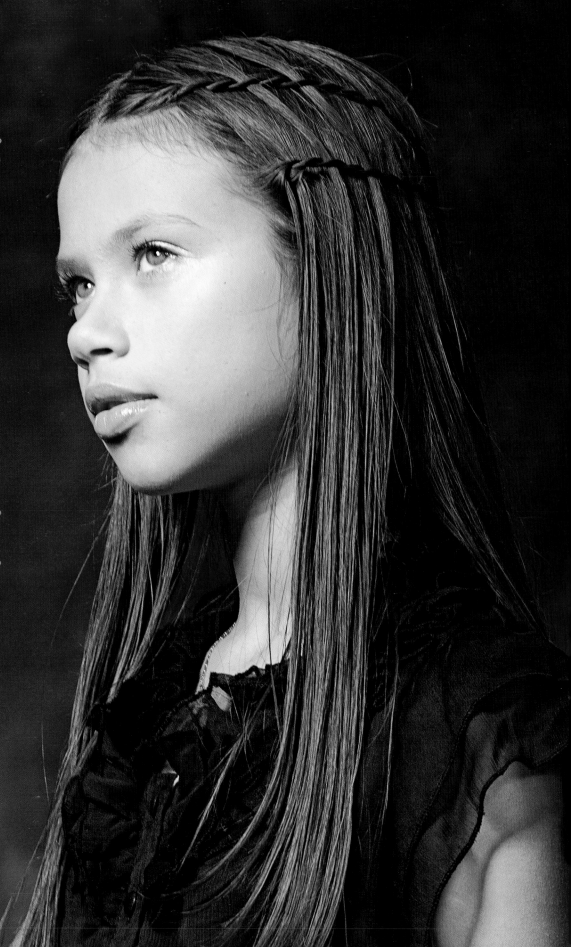

Delicate Double

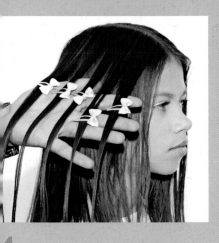

1. Wash and blow dry the hair. Make a middle part from the brow to the nape of the head to divide the hair into two even sections. Draw out several sections of hair on one side of the part and secure each section with a small hair clip.

2. Grasp two small sections of hair at the hairline.

3. Twist each section around itself and then bring the top section over the bottom section to make an X.

4. Grasp the first section of hair that you secured in Step 1 and place it between the two sections of hair forming the X.

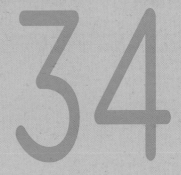

1

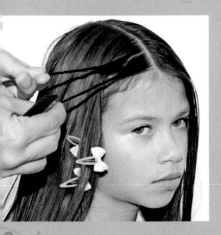

2

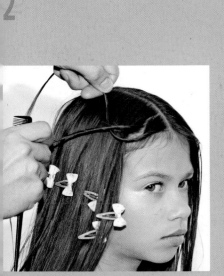

3

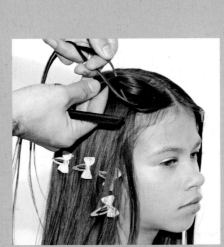

4

Make the most of straight hair by using it to create this dainty double-braided design. It's a simple technique that looks simply lovely.

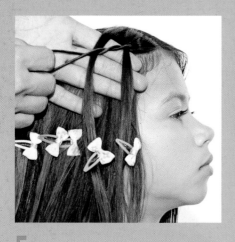

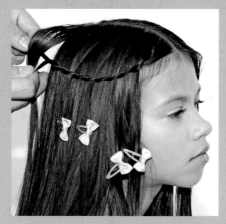

5 **6**

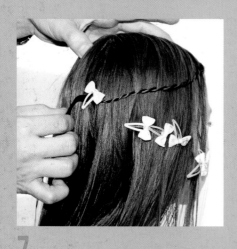

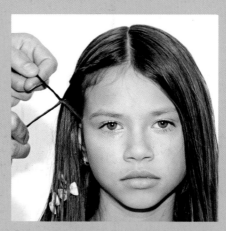

7 **8**

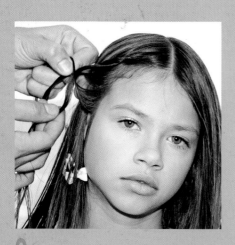

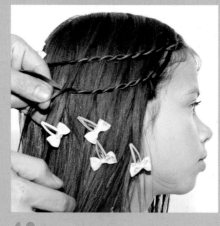

9 **10**

5. Twist this section of hair into the twisted sections and then let it hang loose, leaving the hair clip at the end. Continue drawing the two main twisted sections of hair towards the back of the head. These sections should look a bit like a twisted rope.

6. Grasp the next section of hair that you secured in Step 1. Twist it into the rope of hair and then let it hang loose. Draw the rope of twisted hair backwards and then integrate the next section of hair into it in the same manner. Repeat this technique until you've twisted all the pinned sections of hair into the rope.

7. Secure the end of the rope at the back of the head with a hair clip. Don't remove the hair clips from the bottom of each section of hair.

8. Grasp two small sections of hair at the hairline, below the sections you used to make the first twisted rope.

9. Twist each section around itself and then twist them together to make an X.

10. Grasp the first section of hair that you secured in Step 1 and place it between the two sections of hair forming the X. Twist the hair into the X and then let it hang loose. Continue drawing the rope of hair backwards, twisting in all the sections of hair that you twisted into the first rope to make a second twisted rope.

11. When all the sections have been twisted in, pin the ends of the two twisted ropes together at the back of the head.

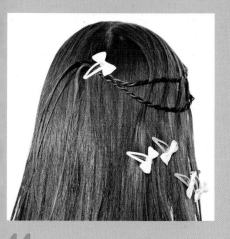

11

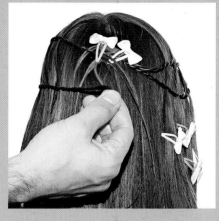

12

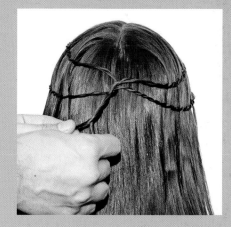

13

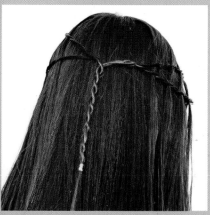

14

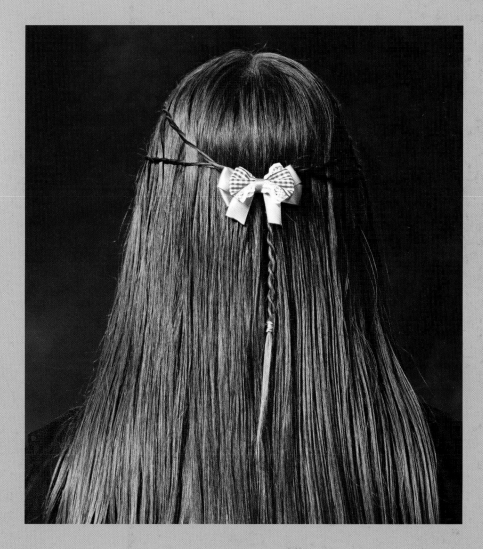

12. Repeat this process on the other side of the head and then pin the ends of all four twisted ropes together.

13. Remove the hair clips on both sides of the head.

14. At the back of the head, twist together the twisted sections to create a rope of hair hanging down the back of the head. Secure with a hair elastic. Add a bow or hair accessory at the top of the rope to finish it off. Mist with holding spray.

Index

Acknowledgments

Monmila Victoria
http://monalina.com
page 24

Style Therapy
www.styletherapy.co.il
pages 20, 44, 92, 120, 124, 136

Sweet Girl Shop
www.sweetgirlshop.co.il
pages 8, 12, 16, 28, 52, 61, 64, 80, 96, 104, 128, 132, 140